FIT
TO EXERCISE

FIT
TO EXERCISE

PROFESSOR EDMUND J. BURKE, Ph.D.

ASSOCIATE PROFESSOR, SPRINGFIELD COLLEGE,
SPRINGFIELD, MASSACHUSETTS

DR JOHN H. L. HUMPHREYS, Ph.D.

PRINCIPAL LECTURER, CARNEGIE SCHOOL OF
PHYSICAL EDUCATION & HUMAN MOVEMENT
STUDIES, LEEDS POLYTECHNIC

FOREWORD BY DR RON HILL, M.B.E.

PELHAM BOOKS
LONDON

First published in Great Britain by
Pelham Books Ltd
44 Bedford Square
London WC1B 3DU
March 1982
Second Impression August 1982

Burke, Edmund J.
    Fit to exercise.
    1. Exercise — Physiological effect
    I. Title   II. Humphreys, John H.L.
    612'.76   QP301

    ISBN 0 7207 1224 6

Typeset by Cambrian Typesetters, Hants
Printed by Hollen Street Press, Slough and
bound by Dorstel, Harlow

CONTENTS

ACKNOWLEDGEMENTS

The authors and publishers are grateful to the following for permission to use copyright material in this book: pages 120 and 121 (tables 10.1 and 10.2) from *The Aerobics Way* by Kenneth H. Cooper, M.D., M.P.H. Copyright © 1977 by Kenneth H. Cooper, reprinted by permission of the publisher, M. Evans and Company Inc., New York 10017; pages 123 and 125 (tables 10.3, 10.4 and 10.6) from *Health and Fitness Through Physical Activity* by Jack H. Wilmore and Samuel M. Fox III Copyright © 1978 by John Wiley & Sons Inc., reprinted by permission of the publisher; page 124 (table 10.5) from *Nutrition, Weight Control and Exercise* by F. Katch and W. McArdle Copyright © 1977 by Houghton Mifflin Company, reprinted by permission of the publisher; pages 134–159 from *Nutritive Value of Foods* U.S.D.A. Home and Garden Bulletin No. 72, 1970, reproduced by permission of the U.S. Dept. of Agriculture; pages 160–162 from *Guidelines for Graded Exercise Testing and Exercise Prescription*, American College of Sport Medicine, Lea and Febiger, Philadelphia 1975.

Illustrations are reproduced by permission of the following: page 33 from *Towards an Understanding of Human Performance* ed. E.J. Burke Copyright © 1980 Mouvement Publications, reprinted by permission of the publishers; pages 57, 58, 61, 94 and 95 from *Prevention of overuse injuries in the distance runner* published in *Relevant Topics for Athletic Training* by K. Scriber and E.J. Burke (eds) Copyright © 1978 Mouvement Publications, reprinted by permission of the publishers; pages 81 to 85 from *Scientific Principles and Methods of Strength Fitness* 2/E by John P. O'Shea Copyright © 1976, Addison-Wesley, Reading, Massachusetts, reprinted with permission; page 78 Mini Gym, Inc., Lexington; page 104 the Mayo Clinic.

With the exception of the photograph on page 78, the photographs are by Gordon Willcock.

FOREWORD BY DR RON HILL, M.B.E.

For 26 years I have been a runner. My training log records over 92,000 miles of training and racing.

For sixteen years I have run every day without missing. Most of these years I was running to try to excel in competition and I won some good races. Now I hardly ever win, but still I continue to run daily. It makes me feel good both physically and mentally. My daily runs are a barometer of how my body is performing and I intend to run until the day I die.

This book sets out admirably why I should feel so good through exercise, and I particularly enjoyed the chapters on evolution and human physiology which put into perspective man's place in time and the need to keep our bodies tuned to what they are supposed to be in a rapidly changing world.

Two areas of possible deficiency in my own physical fitness as defined here are indicated in the chapters on strength and flexibility. My running, which is mainly aerobic, keeps me feeling fine; however, probably one day I will find the time or realise the need to do some stretching and possibly use some weights, when I will pick up this volume again.

PREFACE

This book is meant to be about exercise and you. Your body is the only possession you truly own. We think exercise makes your body a nicer thing to have around! Undoubtedly you are at least mildly interested in exercise. You probably fill one of three categories:

a) You are currently exercising regularly and like exercise books.

b) You used to play sports and want to 'get back in shape'.

c) You have rarely been involved in any systematic exercise programme and/or you certainly haven't done too much in recent years — you're curious.

The topics which we are going to be dealing with should interest each of you. That's certainly our goal!

In assigning writing duties for this book the authors decided to take primary authorship for individual chapters based upon their interests and availability. E.J.B. was the one with the most free time and the decision was made to assign him six chapters (1 to 5 and 8). J.H. had the primary authorship of four chapters (6, 7, 9 and 10). The authors communicated regularly and each accepts full responsibility for the content of the complete book.

The general topic of 'exercise and the body' is not one about which all scientists agree. Furthermore, almost everyone has personal opinions concerning exercise; we certainly do. In writing this book we are attempting to blend a consensus of scientific opinion with our personal experiences. The intent was to make the book both informative and a motivator for you to join us in exercise.

We would like to mention everyone who has had a role in the formulation of this book but that would be impossible. Instead we will mention a few and thank all those whom we failed to mention. We wish to thank Mr Clive Bond, head of Carnegie School of Physical Education and Human Movement Studies, Leeds Polytechnic, Leeds for making it possible for us to work together in the winter and spring of 1979. E.J.B. will always be grateful to Drs Richard Berger, B. Don Franks and Ray Martinez who helped turn a basketball coach into an exercise scientist. The book was clearly improved by the editorial assistance and helpful suggestions of Barbara Adams at Ithaca College, Ithaca, New York.

A special word of thanks should also go to the researchers, many of whom are listed in our list of further reading, for their efforts which made this book possible.

Edmund J. Burke
Springfield College
Massachusetts

John Humphreys
Carnegie School of Physical Education
and Human Movement Studies
Leeds Polytechnic

September 1981

CHAPTER 1

INTRODUCTION

Exercise can and should be a regular part of your life. We are convinced of it.

We could simply provide you with a short, practical guide – a few pictures of warm-up exercises, suggestions about how far and how fast to run, and what kind of running shoes to buy. We intend to do all that but, after years of experience dealing with such diverse groups as world class athletes, the 'average' man or woman in an exercise programme, people of all ages wishing to lose weight, and cardiac patients, we are struck with the universal curiosity of mankind. In this book we are attempting to answer all those questions which we heard on both sides of the Atlantic; to stimulate some new questions; and to ask a few of our own.

A BIOLOGICAL VIEW OF EXERCISE

Of the members of the animal kingdom, only humans have the abilities needed for self-analysis. Only humans ask questions like: 'Who am I?' 'How did I get here?' 'How can I improve myself?' Our central nervous system – the medium for such thoughts – is complex beyond even our own imagination. It is truly what makes us human. However, the brain, which is responsible for our consciousness, does not operate in a closed environment.

The French physiologist, Claude Bernard, was among the first scientifically to recognize the continuity of the entire organism. At the turn of the century he anunciated his principle, the *milieu interieur.* He explained that our body is a highly liquid (up to eighty per cent water) environment in which every cell is in physical communication with every other cell.

Very recent discoveries have shown that all cells in the body are also tied together through heredity. The structures of the cell which pass certain characteristics from generation to generation are the genes. After the union of a woman's ovum and a man's spermatozoum, the cells of the offspring reproduce, based upon the same genetic information. Each human being is, therefore, conceived with a computer programme that works in every cell of the body!

It is now known that this computer programme is run by a very complex protein macromolecule in the genes – DNA (deoxyribonucleic acid). We are the latest recipients of a line of DNA which has passed in our family tree from generation to generation. And the information we receive at conception is considerable – some have estimated that hundreds of books of information were available in our 'original cell'.

DNA represents a history of humanity. In some, as yet mysterious, way it tells us how to survive within our environment. Since humans, for much of their history, have been hunters and foragers, activities requiring constant use of the muscles of the body, DNA must be saying something like: 'Exercise, it's good for you.' We'll amplify this point later.

Mind and Body

Goethe once said that, 'everything has been thought of before, the difficulty is to think of it again.' The concept that the mind and body need to work in harmony has been a consistent theme of great thinkers through the centuries. From Plato[1] to Galen[2], from Milton[3] to Rousseau[4], critical thinkers have expressed the feeling that the mind and body must function harmoniously or the individual diminishes by the malfunction of either. It is this theme which we wish to expand in this book. Exercise as a means of enhancing the physical aspect of humanity has to make life fuller – has to improve the quality of life.

THE 'PHYSICAL' AND THE HUMAN EXPERIENCE

Because of our unique combination of heredity and environment we are, each of us, truly individuals. The possibility of genetic variation

[1] Plato, 4th century B.C.: 'Then send them to the master of gymnastics in order that their bodies may better minister to the virtuous mind.'
[2] Galen, 2nd century B.C.: 'Therefore that form of exercise is recommended which contributes to the health of the body and to the harmonious functioning of the parts and to the strength of the soul.'
[3] John Milton (1608–1674): 'Physical training was to keep youth healthy, nimble, strong, and well in health . . . make them grow large and tall, and to inspire them with a gallant and fearless courage, which will turn into a native and heroic valour.'
[4] Jean Rousseau (1712–1778): 'It is a lamentable mistake to imagine that bodily activity hinders the working of the mind, as if these two kinds of activity ought not to advance hand in hand and as if the one were not intended to act as a guide to the other.'

approaches infinity and no one could ever have the identical environment of another. Many psychologists believe that it is the interaction of the environment and heredity which is the most crucial determinant of behaviour, i.e., it is not one or the other but the timing of heredity and environmental manifestations which have the greatest impact upon the development of the individual.

Almost by definition, individuality assures inequality. We are most certainly not created equal. But, as the Christian Bible points out, each is born with certain talents capable of being multiplied. Perhaps, in this book, we are intimating that quality of life is somehow tied in with an expansion of one's available hereditary characteristics. Call it happiness, competence, self-satisfaction, or self-actualization, the nature of the human condition is to strive for something extra in life. And we believe that exercise is an available extra, missing in the lives of many.

A useful model for an analysis of human experience has been proposed by Professor Tom Evaul of Temple University. He has identified five dimensions of the human being: physical, emotional, social, intellectual and spiritual.

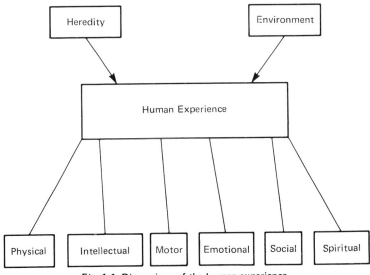

Fig. 1.1 Dimensions of the human experience

Figure 1.1 is a slight modification of Evaul's original model — we have added a 'motor' category. Although each of these categories is different and independent, they develop in one intact human being. They are not exclusive, one of the other. Indeed, this book is devoted

13

partially to the principle that to develop one of these abilities — the physical — is to assist in the development of the others. This relation, between the physical and the other categories from Evaul's model, will be discussed in the rest of this chapter.

Physical

The 'physical' component of human experience — physical fitness or 'being fit' — implies a set of measurable characteristics which have implications for the overall health and sense of well-being of the individual. The 'physical' refers specifically to the efficiency of the heart and lungs, the ability of the joints to move freely, a taut, well-defined musculature, and an absence of unnecessary fat. The 'physical' also has implications for such abstractions as self-esteem and self-confidence. Physical fitness is achieved through a steady, systematic regimen of proper and prudent exercise. In chapters 4, 5, 6 and 7 we will be describing such exercises in great detail. For now it will suffice to say that exercise is an important key to the 'physical'.

Intellectual

Intelligence refers to the capacity of the central nervous system (CNS) to store, classify, and later associate facts and information. We plan, we remember, we experiment, we dream and we create. Above all, we are curious and capable of abstract thought. Intelligence (or lack of it) clearly has a significant impact upon one's life.

Although a frequently used word, 'intelligence' is at present a poorly understood construct. It may generally be possible to recognize individuals high or low in intelligence, but it is very doubtful if the ability can objectively be measured. The I.Q. tests presently available may be classified broadly as environmental achievement tests.

The reason for difficulty in measuring intelligence is that its underlying mechanisms are found in the cerebral cortex. With over ten billion neurons, most with thousands of points of attachment (synapses) there is unbelievable potential for variation and complexity. And, as if the live brain was not already difficult enough to study, neurologists describe it as having the consistency of pudding. To paraphrase the eminent neurophysiologist, John Eccles, our knowledge of how the CNS works is roughly equivalent to the knowledge Columbus would have had if he had wanted to go to the moon! We simply do not have a clue about the underlying physiological mechanism which mediates such human abilities as creativity, problem solving, acquisition and retention of knowledge, mechanical and quantitative abilities, and spatial awareness.

Recently, scientists have learned a few facts which may prove useful in future explanations of brain function. At birth the brain has immense capacity for growth. Therefore, early education is probably very important. We also know that early stimulation — love and affection — seems to be a factor in brain development. Lack of brain development can sometimes be attributed to inadequate pre- and post-natal nutrition.

The centres in the brain which manage and coordinate our muscular actions are very near — anatomically — to the centres for feeling and thinking. It is certainly possible that overlap exists between the motor centre and the association centres. It follows therefore that regular exercise may help in the development of unrelated capacities. We may sometime find a physiological correlate for the feeling: 'I think more clearly when I'm exercising regularly.'

The brain is characterized by its apparent continuity of function. It seems to act as one smoothly functioning, fully integrated computer. And since billions of cells in the motor cortex are given to the regulation of muscular activity it follows that if one part of the brain is little used the entire brain may be adversely affected.

The brain's continuity of function is also of interest when we consider the important influence of lower brain centres on the thinking part of the brain — the cortex. Paul MacLean of the Laboratory of Brain Evolution and Behaviour of the U.S. National Institute of Mental Health has hypothesized a 'Triune brain' model. With evolution we have developed new 'layers' of the brain, keeping the older layers as we build newer ones. He calls the oldest part of the brain the R-complex for its origins in our reptilian past. The next centre is the Limbic system. The highest centres of the brain are found in the cortex — the evolutionary step which has made us distinctly different from other animals.

The lower brain centres regulate such automatic functions as heart rate, respiration, and temperature regulation. They also give us feedback concerning appropriate human behaviour such as eating, sleeping and sexual activities.

In discussing the influence of the Triune brain on human behaviour, Carl Sagan in *Dragons of Eden* reminds us of Plato's metaphor of a charioteer trying to control two powerful horses. In one part, our brain is capable of planning, thought, abstraction, of conscious action. But this same brain is under the influence of lower brain centres, millions of years older. Could it be one of its functions to reward systematic muscular exercise habits with good body feelings — a tingling sense of being alive?

Motor

The human body is able to perform motor skills involving incredibly complex integration of both muscle and nervous system. The balance and grace of the gymnast, the agility of the football striker, the co-ordination of the tennis player are but a few examples of the display of motor ability.

This display of motor ability has root in our distant past and in our present culture. We are the latest in a long chain of humans who, through cleverness and skill, have survived against improbable odds. It may be argued that most sports skills are modern day reenactments of primitive hunting. Rugby, with its emphasis on speed, strength, and physical manhandling of the opponent; soccer, with its required teamwork and speed; cricket, with its gestures of throwing and 'clubbing' — all have a modern manifestation of hunting skills. It must be added, however, that the precise nature of the sport played has cultural implications. The American football player would be playing rugby had he been British. Some individuals, because of certain hereditary factors, will always be drawn to sport; the specific sport to which they are drawn is based on culture.

The physical is a prerequisite for motor fitness. Poor aerobic power, lack of flexibility and strength, and excess fat are all inconsistent with success in sport.

The argument here is not that everyone should be drawn to sport. For those with the 'right parents', sport can be an enjoyable and meaningful part of their life — a means toward self-actualization. For others, sport can only have implications for failure. This is not a book about being 'athletic'; not everyone can be successful in sport. Other factors besides the physical (hunting), such as cleverness and skill of hand, have also influenced the evolution of our bodies. Our position is that everyone can achieve the levels of physical fitness needed for his or her health (see chapter 4). We believe that happiness and self-actualization are possible without being an athlete, but very difficult without adequate physical fitness.

Emotional

Our emotions include human drives such as fear, anger and love. We know that these are controlled by centres in the brain which are among the oldest on the evolutionary scale. The 'emotional' is, then, independent of cold, rational, conscious, logic.

The 'emotional' is especially difficult to define. It may simply be an ability to control our emotions within the standards of society. We all know those who 'lose control' of their emotions and those who seem to be 'under control'.

Several factors may help make a case for exercise and the physical as an adjunct in shaping and controlling our emotions. When the individual is under emotional stress, either chronic or acute, the brain signals for the production of the catecholamines. These substances, commonly termed adrenaline, cause a heightened stimulation which results in such peripheral responses as increased heart rate, higher blood pressure, and perhaps a heightened sense of awareness — anxiety. A systematic, prudent programme of exercise may be of benefit since these catechol-amines are used as a fuel, that is, burned up, during exercise. There is a clear physiological basis for a relaxation in tension as a result of exercise. Indeed those who have taken up jogging in the middle of the day have found a remarkable improvement in their afternoon work output.

Very recent research has pointed to another possible benefit of exercise. We now know that the brain has the ability to secrete power-ful morphine-like chemicals (proteins) called endorphins. They are usually secreted under conditions of stress. As may be expected, they serve the function of combating pain. Dr Richard Thompson of the University of California at Irvine has recently speculated that these biochemicals may be responsible for the 'high' described by many exercisers. He goes further to say that such natural 'highs' might be ideal in dealing with depression. This might explain the 'pick-me-up' effect of exercise.

Social
Social drives arise from the need of humans for cooperation — a survival mechanism. Most people feel a need to be part of a group. A possible cause for the decision of some to become loners is the 'defence mechan-ism' described by Freud. The boy who is laughed at for letting the soccer ball go through his legs or the girl who is last to be chosen for the volleyball team may develop a hatred for sport.

Examples of interaction between the 'physical' and 'social' are numerous. Individuals with similar interests in certain types of sport often come together in formal social arrangements.

Even the most important of social contracts — marriage — is often influenced by the mutual interest or lack of interest in the physical. Marriage counsellors frequently discuss the problems which ensue when one of the marriage partners lets him or herself 'go to pot'. Fear of loss of love is certainly one source of motivation for participation in exercise programmes. Mrs Millie Cooper, wife of the famed fitness expert, Dr Kenneth Cooper, publicly describes her reasons for beginning an exercise programme — among the most important being that she didn't want there to be 'another Mrs Cooper'.

The relationship between the physical and sexual relations must also be noted. Dr Moshe Feldenkrais, in his book *Body and Mature Behaviour*, has drawn an elaborate causal connection between the toned, muscular body and healthy human sexual function. Indeed, biologists have recently measured significant increases in the male sex hormone, test-osterone, in regularly exercising men.

Spiritual
One of the common forms of the human experience, across cultures,

is the establishment of a personal code of ethics. Each of us, implicitly or explicitly, determines his or her balance of personal needs and aspirations versus the needs and aspirations of society. Many would argue that the establishment of such a code is a developmental process.

The Swiss psychologist, Jean Piaget, has hypothesized that the individual gradually develops rules of behaviour based upon individual and social needs. These rules are developed contingent upon and in concert with the development of intelligence. Earlier, Freud argued that the development of morality is based upon early conditions of sexual deprivation. If these theorists are correct, then ethics and morality are developing with, and partially as a function of, the development of the physical — every cell in the body is in communication with every other.

The physical and its development through movement experiences account for numerous human interactions. On the playing fields, is it the game or is winning everything? Do we knock the other person down or do we give everyone a chance at the ball? How do we react to winning? To losing? How does our view of our body coincide with societal values? Do we see a connection between exercise and our body? Who are we?

The personal decisions balancing personal and societal needs almost certainly involve a gradual coming to know who we are. Our view of our body relative to our perception of society's view of our body must have some influence upon our establishment of a code of ethics.

SUMMARY

It is an old, if trite, axiom that we never appreciate our health until it is lost. To that we might add that you can never fully appreciate how good you can feel — the state of positive health — until you take part in a systematic, carefully planned exercise programme.

We must be cautious in our promises, however. Exercise and the development of the physical is not the panacea for all (or even most) of the problems of the human condition. It is only one of several dimensions of the human experience. Undertaken intelligently, systematically and prudently, exercise is one of the good habits which can improve the quality of your life.

CHAPTER 2

BORN TO EXERCISE

A comprehensive scientific analysis of muscular exercise is incomplete without at least a brief search for the origin of our body. Who are we? Where did we come from? How did we come to develop this massive central nervous system? And lest we forget that this is a book about the benefits of exercise: how did muscular exercise affect our development?

Evidence from early cave art suggests that humans have been asking questions like these for thousands of years. Indeed, one of the clear distinguishing characteristics between us and the other advanced animals is our ability to digress from matters of survival – such as eating and mating – for periods of introspection. The human mind has erected great cathedrals, produced magnificent sculpture, and invented music, all in an introspective attempt at discovering who we are and why we are. Lewis Thomas, in his brilliant collection of essays *The Medusa and the Snail*, has said, 'Any species capable of producing, at this earliest juvenile stage of its development, almost instantly after emerging on the earth by any evolutionary study – the music of Johann Sebastian Bach – cannot be all bad.'

Human beings are the ultimate result of over three billion years of life on earth. The accurate, chronological history of our species is of course lost forever, but anthropologists can, based upon certain types of information, make informed hunches concerning our origins.

To understand ourselves fully it is essential that we come to terms with the biological influences in our lives. Although the idea is difficult to discuss in an objective, unemotional way, many biologists would argue that humans have evolved in a father/mother-son/daughter progression from primitive one-celled bacteria. We are the product of a very long period of evolution.

EVOLUTION

The basic theory of evolution proposed by Charles Darwin and Alfred

Russel Wallace, in their joint paper to the Linnean Society in 1859, remains remarkably intact after tens of thousands of subsequent observations and experiments. The theory is as follows: Living organisms contain reproducible characteristics which are passed from generation to generation. Within any species there is an immense diversity of characteristics. But only those which provide an advantage in the battle for survival are retained. Individuals with characteristics appropriate for survival within a given environment live long enough to reproduce, thus retaining the favourable characteristics for the species. Individuals with characteristics unfavourable for survival tend not to live long enough for reproduction, and thus these characteristics tend to die out.

Characteristics such as skin colour, height, visual acuity, blood type, etc., are passed from generation to generation by DNA. Very occasionally, a gene will spontaneously change in some way and this change is called a mutation. These mutations are usually unfavourable to the species (breeding group). Only very rarely does a mutation confer an advantage in survival and, when it does, this characteristic will be selected for inclusion in the species. This is natural selection.

Change within a species is very slow and from species to species, even slower. Usually millions of years are needed for significant change, but the process can be speeded up in small populations during periods of rapid environmental change.

The history of humans and hominids (pre-humans) has unfolded over the last several million years. There is plenty of room for disagreement within the scientific community concerning such matters as the precise lineage of humans[1], the definition of humankind[2], or even the precise age of the human species. However, a fairly broad distinct pattern of findings permits a more or less clear history. The story which unfolds is based upon several types of evidence, none of which taken by itself could provide a final definitive proof, but which, viewed as a whole, provide for us a rich theory of our fairly recent origins.[3]

SOURCES FOR A HISTORICAL PICTURE OF HUMAN LIFE

One of the most important sources of information about our ancestors comes from the analysis of bones. Under the right conditions, bone can

---

[1] It is unclear for instance whether the Neanderthals and Cro-Magnons were our direct ancestors or rivals whom our ancestors exterminated.

[2] Until recently we thought that only humans made tools and were capable of the use of formal language. The work of primatologists has put both of these theories to rest. Indeed Beatrice and Robert Gardner of the University of Nevada have shown that chimpanzees are capable of vocabularies (using sign language) of 100 to 200 words.

[3] The last several millions of years.

remain intact in a state of fossilization for a remarkable length of time. When bones are uncovered, anthropologists are able to make inferences concerning the nature of early humans based upon structural characteristics. The shape of the foot and leg bones, for example, can tell a scientist a lot about the way in which the individual moved from place to place.

The age of bone may be gauged in several ways. Relative dating can be achieved by correlating the fossil in question with the approximate age of the geological deposit in which the specimen was found. Absolute dating is possible by a molecular method using the known decay rate of isotopes such as carbon 14. At death, this isotope begins to decay; the age of the bone may be estimated based upon the amount of decay. This radio carbon technique is fairly accurate for specimens of less than seventy thousand years old. Older finds may be dated with other techniques based upon similar principles, such as the potassium-argon or uranium-thoriem methods.

Scientists are now experimenting with new and more sophisticated techniques of dating. One is the paleomagnetism technique. The earth's magnetic field has not been stable. From a known sequence of events, age may be assigned based upon the prevailing magnetic orientation of the rocks at the time when the fossil was deposited.

Another method of dating involves the correlation of finds with known climatic events. Over the last two million years (the Pleistocene period — Table 2.1), there has been a series of cold and temperate periods in the northern hemisphere (where most of the anthropological research has been conducted). These climactic changes necessarily affected the animals and plants of the period. For example, in a period of near sub-tropical weather, the elephant once roamed the plains of Europe. Studying the evidence of animal and plant life from a deposit can tell us something about its age.

Other methods for gaining insight into early human patterns of life are available. The artifacts in the vicinity of groups of bones may be examined. It is possible to see a clear pattern in the advancement of tools from a simple smoothed pebble, to hand axes and eventually spears. Evidence from pottery and drawings on the walls of caves provides important clues about the culture of early humans.

We also have the example of the primitive tribes of recent and near recent time. There are scattered tribes in northern Scandinavia, central Africa, Australia, and the islands of the Pacific that live lives very similar to those of their ancestors of several thousand years ago. Through research into their habits, it is possible to make sensible hypotheses about the origins of our own culture and life style.

Finally, there is the new and enormously rich research currently being carried on by the primatologists. Analysis of chimpanzee and rhesus

Table 2.1 An outline of hominid history from a European perspective

Geology	Years ago	European geological periods	Arrival of hominids (man's ancestors or rivals)	Cultural events
Holocene	10,000	Post Glacial		use of metals agriculture
			Cro-Magnons	bow and arrow
Upper Pleistocene		Glaciation		cave painting ritual burial
	100,000	Third Inter-glacial	Neanderthals	
		Glaciation		
Middle Pleistocene	250,000	Second Inter-glacial		
		Glaciation		
			Early Homo Sapiens	
	500,000	First Inter-glacial		fire?
Lower Pleistocene		Glaciation		
	750,000	?		
	1 Million	?		hand axe
	2 Million	?	Homo Erectus	pebble tools
Pliocene	3 Million	?	Homo Habilis	use of bones as tools
	5 Million	?	Australopi-thecus	pre-man stands erect

monkey behaviour provides valuable clues concerning our origins. The work of Jane Goodall in the wilds of Central Africa, and that of Harry Harlow in the more controlled setting of his laboratory at the University of Wisconsin-Madison, have provided information useful in finding out who we are and where we have come from.

The search for our origins has taken place with the assistance of an impressive team of scientists. Biologists, biochemists, and physicists have combined with anthropologists, physicians, and engineers. The story they tell is both fascinating and informative. It is at best difficult, at worst impossible, fully to understand ourselves or our society without reacting to the following story.

OUR NEAREST RELATIVES

Over seventy million years ago mammals first appeared. The first mammals were shrew-like creatures who probably had their origins in the trees. Because of their arboreal existence, they were characterized by excellent vision and a reduced capacity for smell. Over the next twenty-five to thirty million years of evolution their brain grew dramatically. Life in the trees, with every gymnastic swing through space a potential endpoint in evolution, may have served to select a brain where intelligence was of particular value.

Initially the small prosimians, later the monkeys, and finally the apes appeared. The primates of forty million years ago, like those of today, had characteristics which seemed to suit them well for their life in the trees.

Clearly the most important adaptive characteristic of the primates was the increased size of their brain. Another characteristic which may have developed in conjunction with the large brain is the ability of the forearm and hand to work together for grasping, thus making the use of tools possible.

All primates have the characteristic of 'sociability'. They tend to form small units with one male, several females and their immature offspring. Small bands or troops are then formed from these units and led by a dominant male. Relative to other animals, the primates have an exceedingly long period of immaturity, in which it is possible to teach the skills needed for survival. During this period, most young primates spend a lot of time at play, which appears to be a form of mental rehearsal under conditions of comparative safety. Having a wrestling match, for example, does not have the same serious consequences as a fight to the death.

THE HUMAN SPECIES

Primates have existed for about forty million years – humans only about one to five million at the most. Environmental conditions at the end of the Pliocene (see Table 2.1) probably helped to stimulate humans' withdrawal from their arboreal heritage. In central and south Africa, at the end of the Pliocene, there were substantial decreases in temperature and rainfall. There was undoubtedly a breakup of the forest, with subsequent creation of grassy savannahs. The success of primates in numbers may have also driven some out of the trees.

For whatever reason, our ancestors left their former environment, coming to live on or at the edge of the grasslands. Lacking in speed, strength, and other essential skills needed for survival, our ancestors survived and flourished by becoming more clever than the other animals. Life in the open called for a clear selection of the most intelligent. They probably grouped together in small troops; cooperation was essential. Competition, incidentally, is a much newer trait and only occurred as space became limited. But until a few million years ago our ancestors probably lived an existence not unlike today's chimpanzee.

When did our ancestors become human? Needless to say, we don't have the answer to that question. Most physical anthropologists would say that there was no one date. Rather, it is more likely that by a very gradual process, involving several millions of years, the hominids (prehumans), developed the physical and mental characteristics that led to the species we would call homo sapiens.[4]

In 1925, the anthropologist Raymond Dart found the skull of an eight or nine-year-old child in South Africa. The skull, which he called *Australopithecus*, has had immense importance for a study of the history of human life. From the angle of the foramen magnum (the hole at the base of the skull), it was possible to deduce that this individual was walking, at least partially, upright. Later finds of complete sets of bones, including legs and feet, support this conclusion. Dart's australopithecine skull was about two million years old. More recently Richard Leakey and his workers have dated the origin of *Australopithecus* at about five and a half million years.

The evolutionary step of walking upright had important future implications. The hands of *Australopithecus* were now free to make and use tools and weapons. The hominids were in a sense forced to live by their wits. Tools were needed to make up for their obvious physical limitations. And an improved brain power was necessary to construct and effectively use the tools. A gigantic feedback loop — each improvement tended to accentuate the next — was free to unfold. The chain of events has led to us.

---

[4]Most biologists would define a species as a group capable of mating and bearing offspring within itself. Some anthropologists have differentiated intelligent man (homo sapiens) from modern intelligent man (homo sapiens sapiens).

Remains of other types of bipedal hominids have also been found – homo habilis and homo erectus. Their origin and their eventual fate is by no means clear. Were they our ancestors or did we exterminate them?

Compared with *Australopithecus* both of the more recent hominids are characterized by an increasing skull size, a more erect posture and a more complex pattern of living. From their teeth and the nature of their tools we know that the members of homo habilis were meat eaters, but not yet hunters, i.e., they were probably at least partially scavengers living off the 'kills' of other animals while using their ability to grasp sticks and clubs to beat off the other scavengers. The more modern homo erectus spread all over the world – to Java, to Europe, to China, to India. From their tools we know that by one million years ago humans survived by hunting.

For a very, very long time, perhaps several millions of years from the advent of the first hominids, food gathering habits remained approximately the same. Food gathering involved a daily search for fruits, nuts, berries, and other products of the environment which could provide adequate nutrition for survival. This process was inefficient and certainly could not support a very large human population.[5]

As the hominid's brain grew, the complexity of weapons and tools advanced correspondingly. Our human ancestors were becoming aware of new and more efficient methods of survival. Beginning with the eating of the spoils of other animals' prey, progressing to the capture of small animals, eventually the hunting of large animals was initiated – maybe one million years ago.

Large animals clearly provided superior sources of protein and calories, thus making possible the maintenance of larger populations. Hunting dramatically altered the course of mankind. It required aggression, strength, speed, aerobic power (indeed, all of the components of physical fitness described in chapter 4), and cleverness. Natural selection had to provide a species of alert, inventive and physically fit individuals. But cooperation was also essential. In attempting to trap and kill an animal many times the size and strength of a human, individual wants had to give way to the needs of the community. Oral communication and planning were essential. It was necessary to have a more sophisticated culture in which knowledge of where and when to find food, hunting skills, tool and weapon making and hunting strategies were passed from generation to generation. Hunting parties were formed and led by the fittest male. Fitness was probably assessed by brainpower, size, strength,

---

[5]With the exception of the gorilla, man is presently the largest of the primates. Although the gorilla is a true vegetarian it has always been among the least successful of the primates, if success is measured in numbers. It survives only in densely thick jungle areas.

and hunting skill. And there was a need for division of labour along sex lines.

Sex role identification based upon biological considerations has been made for at least the last million years and probably a lot longer. Because of the males' larger size (for forty million years of primate history the largest of the males had their pick of the available females) and strength (the male hormone testosterone gives immense strength advantages), the male was charged with hunting and defending the group against 'outsiders'.

Coincidentally, the development of the human brain was clearly 'locking in' the role of the female. The increasing size of the neonate skull called for an ever widening of the female pelvis[6], which in turn decreased her efficiency in the hunt. The long nine-month gestation period called for the natural selection of greater fat stores in the female, further decreasing her relative ability in the hunt. The increasing complexity of the central nervous system called for longer periods of neonate helplessness — more time was needed for the brain to mature. Breast feeding, and the female's relative inferiority in the hunt, meant that she was assigned the role of caring for the pitifully helpless human neonates. And evolution undoubtedly rewarded the female with special sensations leading to behaviour we may describe as tenderness or affection. Recent research has shown the human infant's need for fondling and touching — for love. Without it, the central nervous system often develops poorly. Selective advantages must have resulted in a feedback loop where the mother[7] not only cared for the young out of necessity but received biological feedback for doing so. Female hormones were surely at least partially responsible for the care and protection of each succeeding 'next generation' of the species.

Both sexes were capable of prodigious amounts of work and therefore needed great aerobic power. While the male hunted, the female and her available immature offspring foraged for nuts and berries in the vicinity of their semi-fixed home. Invention and repair of clothing, cooking, construction of shelters and eventually the maintenance of the hearth were among the many important duties of the female.

During the last several million years, the hunting/gathering life style of our nearest ancestors resulted in a need for travel. The available plants

---

[6] In *Dragons of Eden*, Carl Sagon has noted that to his knowledge human females are alone in the animal kingdom in their agonizing pain at childbirth. Apparently phylogeny has gone as far as it can in widening the female pelvis — a wider pelvis would simply not permit her adequate mobility.

[7] In her suberb text *The Psychology of Women*, Judith Bardwick relays to the reader her own experience as a mid-20s Ph.D. interested in research and the women's movement. But after giving birth to a child, this helpless baby suddenly became the focus of her entire life.

and animals were used up as a region became overpopulated. Although each succeeding generation probably advanced the frontier only a small amount, by one million years ago humans had colonized most of the globe.

The problems of our European ancestors must have led to very trying circumstances indeed. As humans travelled into the Northern Hemisphere, the periods of glaciation called for remarkable abilities in adaptation. Glaciers descended over all Europe and North America as far south as Kansas City for periods sometimes longer than one hundred thousand years. And just to test human capacity for adaptation, the weather would then warm up for periods of ten thousand years. At one point, Europe had a nearly semi-tropical environment with elephants roaming the plains. The warming trends would cause great walls of water[8] to descend, shifting continents, cutting off such home lands of human life as the British Isles. It is possible to imagine a picture of the intelligent, social animal, eking out an existence, surviving against fantastic odds.

For most of human history, the development of technology was pitifully slow. The first tools may have been smoothed pebbles, sticks, and bones. Hand axes and pointed spears evolved. Methods for the construction of semi-permanent shelters and for the making of clothing were important. The harnessing of fire nearly five hundred thousand years ago must have been a major achievement. But all the earlier inventions pale in comparison with the invention of agriculture, which made possible the technological world in which we live. Agriculture permitted humans to make proper use of their massive brain, but it also paved the way for a reduced need of the muscles.

Agriculture was probably begun in the fertile Nile river crescent about ten thousand years ago. The planting and harvesting of wheat meant that humans could rely on a steady yearly supply of food. No longer was life a day-to-day existence. A technological explosion was made possible. The wheat and grain had to be portioned out, making mathematics necessary. Record keeping required writing. Towns began to spring up, bringing merchants and trade. With extra time available, art and music could grow. And of course the riches of some meant that others would kill for them. Wars, first between cities, and then city-states, were a part of mankind.

For us, the implications of technology are many. We live longer than our ancestors. By most standards we live fuller lives; the car, cinema, radio and television see to it that we are constantly stimulated. From a purely biological point of view, our vast increase in population serves to

---

[8]Perhaps these great cataclisms resulted in legends such as Noah and his ark or of the lost city of Atlantis.

validate the importance of technology. However there remains a malaise in the minds of many. Lionel Tiger, Professor of Anthropology at Rutgers University described it well:

> We know that a civilisation based on mass organization has its discontents. Many of us feel unimportant as persons, derive little pleasure from our work and little sense of protection and grace from our widely scattered families. To generate healthy social change in the future, or even to come to terms with what exists in the present, we must lose our blindness to our past. Oddly enough, seeing ourselves as animals may make the future more humane.

Our society has developed into one where the cortex of the brain appears to dominate — maybe it always has, it has been just a matter of degree. However, we should not lose sight of our muscular heritage.

Humans are capable of fantastic feats of physical prowess. Some individuals are capable of nearly continuous runs lasting for days; of short bursts of speeds covering one hundred yards in less than ten seconds; of lifting weights equal to and greater than their own body weights; indeed of lifting their centre of gravity to heights greater than their own. However, no longer are such muscular efforts valuable or necessary for survival — even warfare has been reduced to button pushing. Mostly because of technology, we often complain if we have to walk to a bus. And yet, certainly nothing of significance has happened to our genes in a mere ten thousand years.

A BIOLOGICAL CASE FOR EXERCISE

Based upon the presently accumulated knowledge, a biological hypothesis for exercise, with reasonable chance of being proved, may be made. We begin the deductive process with the premise that a considerable portion of human behaviour is predicated upon genetic information in the DNA or our parents' germ cells. By definition — we are alive against considerable odds — this genetic information has proved useful in the survival of the species. Given the importance of exericse as a means of survival throughout most of the history of the species (or the class), it follows that somewhere in the genetic blueprint is an order to exercise!

The manner in which the genetic command gets translated into human behaviour is largely unknown. It probably works with some interplay between DNA, RNA, enzyme synthesis and the twelve billion neurons of the central nervous system. The hypothalamus is known to be a site of pleasure in the brain. The joy and elation many of us receive

28

from exercise is likely to be centred in this structure. Although the machinery may not be understood for many years, those who exercise regularly test the validity of the hypothesis.

An alternative biological case for exercise is also available. The body is in fact a highly fluid environment where every cell is in communication with every other. While the central nervous system dominates the organism, a very great deal of the work of the body is given over to the flow of materials to and from the muscles (forty per cent of the body by weight). How can the central nervous system responsible for thinking, dreaming, creating, playing, and loving, function at optimal levels in a body where fully forty per cent is left to waste away through neglect? We could of course make the same case for the fitness buff who totally neglects his or her mind. Montaigne said it best: 'It is not a mind, it is not a body that we are training; it is a man, and he ought not to be divided into two parts.'

A FINAL THOUGHT

Most children love to play. They love to run, to hop, to throw, to climb, to skip, to jump. Some would say that in play we see a recapitulation of the early days of humans — preparation for a muscular life of hunting, gathering and preparing for the next generation. Certainly play involving big muscle exercise provides a framework for the healthy development of bone and muscle, and most children derive a great deal of pleasure from it. But what happens in western culture between childhood and adult life that results in reports that less than half of the adults in America engage in any form of exercise — including fifteen minute walks?

One cause may be our glorification of sport and athletes. Our modern athlete tends to be a latter day reincarnation of the great hunter or soldier. In many respects it is only natural that we tend to look up to them. But unlike earlier days, we are only rarely asked to use our own muscles. We sit in stadiums and arenas wildly cheering as, vicariously, we take part on the field of battle. We admire the beautiful bodies of the athletes, while doing nothing for our own.

Only a small number of individuals are born with the combination of abilities needed to be successful in sport. For example, it is a sad commentary that, in America, millions of inner-city youths dream about becoming a professional basketball player, yet only three hundred jobs are available. The odds are only marginally better for British soccer. These sports would be fine if only people would take part without the prospect of external rewards. And yet, most physical education programmes continue to deal primarily with sports such as football and rugby.

In discussing this issue at a recent meeting, a senior officer of the British Sports Council countered the allegation that there should be a drastic change in the nature of physical education in the schools of the West with the statement, 'In England everyone gets plenty of opportunity to play soccer in schools — no problem!' But this is a problem. Very few individuals can be successful at soccer: most fail and some, often those who most need exercise, are laughed at. Even those good enough to play for a school or club frequently stop at twenty-one, with about fifty years of life left to live! It is not inconsistent to be both a strong proponent of sport and a vigorous advocate of physical education for all.

This book is about exercise which does not require you to be an athlete. Indeed, few people can be athletes, but nearly everyone can experience the joy of being physically fit.

CHAPTER 3

OUR BODY AND EXERCISE

Our bodies are marvellous creations of engineering. We have structure (anatomy) and function (physiology) adequate to explore and people the entire planet. No other animal is so adaptable.

Our bodies, like those of other members of the animal kingdom, are machines ideally suited for exercise. Indeed, over seventy per cent of our body is given over to the purpose of movement; thirty to forty per cent to the muscular system, thirty to forty per cent to the bones. In order to gain a greater appreciation of the potential benefits of exercise, we shall analyze the body, and in particular those systems which allow us to do physical work.

OXYGEN FOR EXERCISE

One of the most important developments in the evolutionary process ending in mankind was that of the ability, by one-celled animals, to make use of oxygen from the air in order to do the work of the cell. As a result, far greater amounts of work were possible.

Every cell of our body depends upon adequate supplies of oxygen, i.e., most of the work of the body is done aerobically. For a very short while we can work without oxygen, i.e., anaerobically, as our muscles have a few seconds' worth of oxygen stored. Also, the blood can store about two to five minutes' worth, depending upon the individual. But beyond five minutes — less for some — we cannot survive. We will now examine the systems of the body which have the greatest influence upon the ability to use oxygen.

Respiratory system

The body has developed many mechanisms for the transport and utilization of oxygen (see Figure 3.1). Initially we take in air, which contains about twenty-one per cent oxygen. The air flows through our nose and mouth, down a long system of tubes or canals. At the end of these air passageways are millions of tiny bags of air, the alveoli. Our lungs are little more than air bags expanding and contracting as a result of the muscles which pull on the rib cage. When the muscles of inspiration contract, the consequent pressure differential between the lung air and the atmospheric air causes an air inflow. Likewise, when the respiratory muscles relax, a pressure differential causes an air outflow.

Circulatory system

The circulatory system has two important responsibilities: to provide oxygen and nutrients to the cells of the body; and to remove the waste products of the cell.

We have just described the passage of oxygen from the room air to the tiny, end-point air sacs, the alveoli. Passing by the alveoli are tiny, one-cell thick capillaries which contain blood. The blood travelling to the lungs has come from the right side of the heart and is returning from the working cells. It is oxygen starved and contains relatively high concentrations of the cells' waste product, carbon dioxide.

Most of the oxygen and carbon dioxide is carried by the red blood cells. Because of the impressive binding power of the protein, haemoglobin, contained in the red blood cells, each cell is capable of carrying millions of molecules of oxygen and carbon dioxide. And although there are several million red blood cells, they squeeze, one at a time, through a pulmonary capillary to be filled up, as Dr Kenneth Cooper has suggested, like so many milk bottles in a dairy. As the red blood cell comes near the alveolus, a basic physical process takes place. The oxygen diffuses from the higher concentration of the lungs to the blood, while the carbon dioxide diffuses from the blood into the alveolus. As we exhale, we deposit the carbon dioxide into the air thus freeing the process to continue.

Once the oxygen is in the blood it is transported a few centimetres to the left side of the heart. It enters the left atrium, passes through the mitral valve, and enters the large left ventricle. This left ventricle is a powerful pump capable of prodigious levels of work. In a normal life time the heart pumps out over two hundred million quarts of blood − over forty-three thousand quarts in a day.

During contraction of the heart, the blood is pumped through the aorta, the largest artery in the body. One of the blood's first stops as it travels out to every cell in the body is the heart itself.

Coronary circulation

The heart is a muscle, similar to a thigh or calf muscle. It too needs oxygen in order to contract and therefore is supplied with its own blood vessels called the coronary arteries. These first branches of the

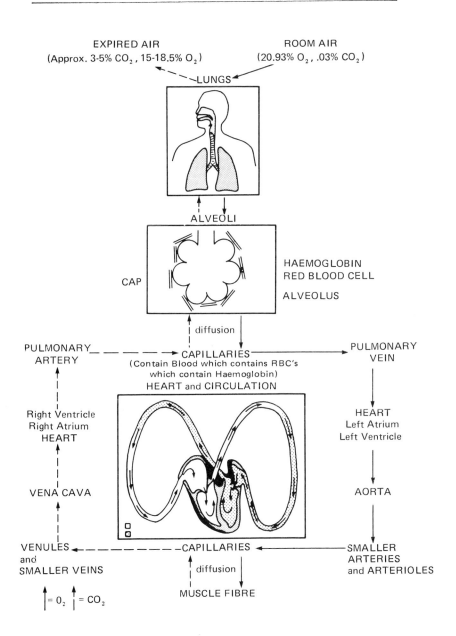

Fig. 3.1 The oxygen and carbon dioxide transport system

aorta are called the right and left coronary arteries (see Figure 3.2). Just as with the lungs, the blood vessels branch and form ever finer tubes ending in the tiniest blood pathways, the capillaries. Blood vessels seem to have the ability to form new branches — extra branches on the 'vascular tree'. These extra blood vessels are called collateral circulation. These new blood vessels are sometimes formed as a result of too little oxygen being available — out of necessity. Alternatively, waves of blood 'gushing' into the area may open dormant vessels. Both conditions occur during 'aerobic' exercises.

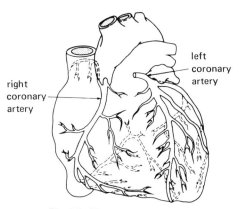

right
coronary
artery

left
coronary
artery

Fig. 3.2   The coronary arteries

Although by no means universally accepted, the possibility that exercise may be of benefit by increasing the blood supply to the heart has been proposed by numerous authorities. If proved, the benefits are obvious. With little collateral circulation, it follows that a blockage[1] will cause a great deal of heart muscle to be without oxygen. A heart attack could be imminent. In the myocardial infarction (heart attack), heart muscle dies as a result of oxygen deprivation. The severity of the heart attack depends upon the amount of heart muscle which dies, which in turn depends upon the amount of heart muscle which was deprived of blood (oxygen). If, as some physiologists have found, the amount of collateral circulation is increased as a result of sound exercise habits, it follows that the potential for a heart attack is diminished. And if a heart attack does occur, almost every cardiologist will testify to the ability of the systematic exerciser to withstand it better than the non-

[1] Perhaps caused by a small blood clot (coronary thrombosis) or by a clogged artery (atherosclerosis).

exerciser. This could be a function of either the extra collateral circulation, or the high quality muscle of the exerciser's heart, or a combination of the two.

Circulation to the muscles

In addition to distributing blood to the heart, the aorta and its tributaries distribute it to all parts of the body: the stomach, intestines, liver, spleen, bone, kidneys, and of course the brain are all users of oxygen. But the prime users of the body's blood are the skeletal muscles. At rest, the muscles use twenty to twenty-five per cent of the body's blood reservoirs, and during exercise the figure rises to ninety per cent. If the muscles are asked to do little or no work (require relatively small quantities of blood), the whole system is bound to suffer.

Muscles

Muscles are usually arranged with two points of connection with bone. Normally one of the bones is fixed or semi-fixed, while the other is movable. When the fibres, which are arranged parallel to the long axis of the muscle, contract, movement occurs.

The muscle fibre consists, in part, of the functional units of the cell, the protein (actin and myosin) molecules. These slide together when energy is available, causing the characteristic firm, taut skeletal muscle. In order for the protein molecules in muscle cells to slide together, they must produce energy from a combination of the food we eat and the oxygen in the air. Both come to the muscle cell through the circulation.

As the blood arrives at the working muscle cell (fibre) in the tiny one-cell thick capillaries, a transmitting substance, myoglobin, passes the needed oxygen to the mitrochondrion – the power plant of the cell. A muscle cell is provided with hundreds of mitrocondria, each with an infinitely complex yet simple and efficient set of mechanisms for the production of energy. The energy produced permits the muscles to contract, resulting in movement. Carbon dioxide produced in the process returns to the blood, resulting in the darker appearance of venous blood.

The veins return the blood to the heart and thence to the lungs with the help of a marvellous adaptation, which enables blood to travel 'up hill'. The inner walls of the veins are provided with one-way flaps which prevent a back flow of blood. As long as there are muscles to squeeze on the veins[2], the blood can only flow in one direction – back to the heart. Thus, we can see how toned, well muscled legs can be of assistance to the heart.

[2] Of course some individuals, such as barbers and dentists, who stand all day for years have severe problems with the return of blood to the heart, resulting in varicose veins.

FUEL FOR EXERCISE

We eat in order to provide the cells with the nutrients and energy[3] needed for work. As food passes from the mouth to the stomach to the intestines, a series of enzymes composed of complex protein molecules act upon the food to reduce it to a simpler form, for example, from starch to glucose. Once in its simplest form, the usable food is passed into the blood stream. The unusable components of food, such as cellulose in apples, are passed out at the end of the digestive tract as the body's waste material. Liquid, high-carbohydrate foods may reach the blood stream as fast as one hour. Solid, 'starchy' carbohydrate meals reach the blood in about two to three hours. Proteins are slower and meals high in fat may take six hours and longer. (For more about these foods see chapter 8.)

Through several research studies we now know that the primary fuels for exercise are the carbohydrates and fats. In short, all-out work, carbohydrates are used exclusively as fuel by the muscles. Less than all-out work, which extends for an hour, relies on an approximately 60:40 ratio of fat and carbohydrates. Longer work calls for an increasing importance of fat as fuel. Although fats are the principal fuel source during prolonged exercise, it should be noted that when carbohydrates are depleted, the individual experiences total fatigue.

HOW YOUR BODY PERFORMS PHYSICAL WORK

Muscular contraction during exercise involves a complex interaction between the nervous and muscular system. Large muscles are composed of bundles of many thousands of individual muscle fibres. The muscle fibre is wrapped; collections of muscle fibres are wrapped in bundles; and the bundles are wrapped in a collection of bundles. The wrapping material is extremely thin and, when it has not been used for a while, it can be easily torn. This is one of the reasons for soreness the day after exercise following a long layoff. It is also a reason for gradually warming up, so that you are less likely to tear this wrapping material of muscle.

Muscle fibres receive their command to contract from the nervous system. Of interest is the fact that muscle fibres receive not only commands to contract but also commands to remain relaxed. Inhibition of the muscle appears to be a safety factor in preventing the muscle from literally 'tearing itself away' from the bone or deep connective tissues. Reduction of inhibiting influences on muscle may be responsible for the reports of mothers lifting cars off their children, or small sailors

---

[3]Oxygen and the end products of our food combine in the mitochondrion to form energy. This is called aerobic metabolism.

throwing four hundred pound bombs over the side of carriers during a fire.

An interesting finding from recent research studies is that the muscle is provided with at least two distinctive types of fibres (cells): 'fast twitch' for all-out contractions; and 'slow twitch' for contractions over a long period of time. The muscles which you use to run have a given percentage of each fibre type and can utilize only the appropriate fibre type for a given activity — while the slow twitch fibres are used extensively in a marathon run, the fast twitch fibres will be used very little and are useful for sprints. Apparently fibre type distribution is controlled by heredity. It would obviously be of benefit to have a high concentration of slow fibres if you wanted to be a successful long distance athlete. Likewise, a high concentration of fast fibres would be needed for success in the 100-yard sprint. This is one of the prime reasons that the famous exercise scientist, Per Olof Astrand of Sweden, points out that if you want to be a great athlete you must be very careful in 'picking your parents'.

EXERCISE CONTROL MECHANISMS

Exercise requires a complex system of control mechanisms involving certain glands, and the circulatory, respiratory, musculo-skeletal, and nervous systems. All work in harmony to permit the full functioning of our muscles.

Simply thinking about exercise brings into play a series of mechanisms which result in supplying the working muscles with oxygen and essential nutrients, while providing a means of ridding the body of the muscle's waste products. The process begins in the brain where signals may be sent to various control points in the body. Prior to exercise, the heartbeat quickens and the breathing becomes deeper and more rapid. Essential muscle blood vessels are expanded while blood vessels to 'non-essential' areas, such as the stomach and kidneys, are constricted. Constriction of the veins results in an increased flow of blood back to the heart. With the onset of exercise, the pancreas and adrenal glands secrete the hormones glucagon and epinephrine, respectively, which mobilize the sugar and fat stores for ready access by the muscles. As the amount of oxygen in the blood drops and as the waste products of the muscle, such as carbon dioxide, increase in the blood stream, control mechanisms are signalled in the lower brain centres which cause the respiratory muscles to work harder and also the heart to beat faster with greater strength. The maximum amount of blood pumped by the heart with each beat, termed the stroke volume, reaches a maximum at fairly low levels (40–60% of $\dot{V}O_2$ max or heart rates of about 120–140) of exercise. It is for this reason that we recommend submaximal exercise that you might describe as 'somewhat hard'. Work that is 'hard' does little extra for the heart (see Table 3.1).

Oxygen is carried in the blood principally by the haemoglobin. Because of its iron atoms, haemoglobin has an amazing ability to carry oxygen. Some authorities have estimated that without haemoglobin it would take three hundred pounds of blood to carry the oxygen needed at rest! Haemoglobin becomes almost fully saturated (ninety-seven per cent) with oxygen at normal air pressure. As it travels through the arterial system, haemoglobin gives up little of its oxygen but it does so freely at the capillary site.

Perception of Effort*	Heart Rate**	Stroke Volume (Blood pumped by heart with each beat)
Light	100	60% of Max
Fairly Light	120	80% of Max
Somewhat Hard	150	Max
Hard	170	Max
Very Hard	185	Max

* During a run of various speeds
** Assumes a thirty-year old individual who exercises aerobically three times per week.

Table 3.1 Perception of effort in relation to heart rate and stroke volume

The pattern of blood flow during exercise is rather interesting. With the onset of exercise there is a widening of blood vessels serving the muscles, resulting in a substantial increase in blood flow to the muscles. Correspondingly, there is a narrowing of blood vessels to the stomach, kidneys and other 'less essential' (to exercise) areas. Thus the body, through signals from the brain, is being readied for 'flight or fight'. Blood flow to the skin is also increased as the blood is brought near the body's surface for the purpose of cooling. But as exercise proceeds to near maximum levels, the blood flow to the skin is actually reduced, as the muscles take all available blood. This results in a characteristic paleness or pallor. It is a condition which we do not recommend.

As exercise proceeds there is a decrease in the fluid portion of the blood, as the blood plasma is changed to sweat and transported to the surface of the body. It is of some interest that sweat contains lower concentrations of salt and other minerals (electrolytes) than does the blood. It is therefore critical that we replace the water lost, especially on hot days[3]. Exercise on cold days presents problems only in the worst of weather[4].

THE NATURE OF FATIGUE

Assuming that you are working well within your ability to provide oxygen to the muscles, you should be able – after a progressive training period – to work comfortably for several minutes, even to an hour or more. We must emphasize the matter of progressive training. Start slow! If you have not exercised for a while, your system simply may not be used to providing large amounts of oxygen to the muscles. Neither are the muscles capable of using large amounts of oxygen.

What causes the fatigue seen in distance runners following a race? There are several possible answers. They may be out of carbohydrates which are needed by the brain. They may have lost too much water or salt. Or their body temperature may be too high. The reason for their fatigue greatly differs from that of the beginning exerciser. It is unlikely that the above reasons would ever affect the novice runner. He simply does not run long enough. The main reason for fatigue in the recently sedentary individual is the build-up of lactic acid caused by a system that cannot supply and/or use oxygen. This is dangerous enough to remind you once again – start slow!

THE TRAINING EFFECT

Several alterations occur in your body as you improve your ability to exercise, i.e. you are running farther and faster with no more difficulty. We refer to these changes or adaptations as the 'training effect'.[5]

The person in the trained state is usually characterized by a high per cent lean body mass and a low per cent body fat. Individuals in the trained state commonly have connective tissue, such as ligaments and

[3]Temperature regulation becomes a problem when the temperature rises above 80°F with the humidity above eighty per cent. Under these conditions it is important not to overdo exercise and to drink plenty of fluids.

[4]Exercise on cold days presents a different problem as the skin blood vessels are constricted in order to retain heat. Exercise is safe as long as clothing is adequate – wool is best. Only when the wind chill factor dips below 0°F is there a danger of frostbite – where the skin blood vessels constrict to such an extent that patches of skin change colour. Also, do not run into the wind when the temperature is 20°F or less. The cold presents no danger to lungs as the respiratory system is remarkable for its ability to warm cold air to desirable temperatures.

[5]The technical and somewhat complex nature of the known human adaptations to exercise precludes a full and complete description of the 'training effect' in the present volume. The interested reader is directed to the volume by Astrand and Rodahl (1977).

tendons which are thicker, larger and stronger than normal.

Training results in several changes in the lungs' capacity for processing air. The trained individual usually needs a lot less air to do a given amount of work. At the other end of the continuum, we have all seen the individual who has to catch his/her breath after walking up a flight of stairs. This is a good sign of low aerobic power and a poor state of training. With physical training, one can process more air, both in one breath and over many breaths (per minute), if called upon to do so. And at the cellular level, the tiny little air sacs of the lungs, alveoli, are served with more blood resulting in less wasted lung space.

Relative to overall body health, perhaps the most important aspect of the training effect is associated with the beneficial adaptations in the circulatory system. The trained heart is usually larger and stronger. But most importantly, it is provided with greater numbers of blood vessels. The net effect is to increase the amount of blood pumped with each heart beat. As a result, both at rest and in response to a specific amount of exercise, the number of heart beats needed is reduced. Prior to the onset of your training programme, be sure to get an accurate count of your resting heart rate. One of the surest results of an exercise programme is that the resting heart rate will be decreased.

Several other beneficial changes have also been found in the circulatory system as a result of exercise. Blood vessels all over the body and especially those serving the muscles may increase in size, number and elasticity. These changes in conjunction with a loss of needless blood vessels to excess fat (as fat is lost) often but not always result in a decrease in blood pressure.

The red blood cells usually become more numerous as does the oxygen carrying capacity of each red blood cell, resulting in an improved oxygen delivery system to the heart and skeletal muscles.

The combined effect of all these adaptations results in an overall improvement in the individual's maximal ability to use oxygen during heavy work, the $\dot{V}O_2$ max. Improvement in $\dot{V}O_2$ max of approximately 20 to 25 per cent may be expected with eighteen months to two years of continuous training (assuming a non-trained state at the onset). Much higher percentage improvements are possible in very sedentary people or those with certain forms of heart disease. Interestingly, many years of training do not result in yearly improvements of $\dot{V}O_2$ max. Everyone appears to have some hereditarily controlled maximum level. What long periods of training do accomplish is to permit the athlete to work for longer periods at higher percentages of $\dot{V}O_2$ max, e.g. the untrained individual might become fatigued working for 5 to 10 minutes at 75 per cent of $\dot{V}O_2$ max; in contrast, the same marathon runner can run for two hours at 90 per cent of $\dot{V}O_2$ max! The precise mechanisms for this adaptation are presently unknown.

SUMMARY

In this chapter we have made a brief attempt at summarizing the several anatomical and physiological factors which affect your ability to exercise. In order for muscles to contract, they need energy from food (that's not much of a problem for the body as most people have plenty of energy stored in fat) and oxygen (that's a considerable problem for the sedentary untrained body). The oxygen is transported in the blood which is pumped to the muscle cells by the heart. To be able to use a lot of oxygen, therefore, implies a healthy heart and circulatory system.

To build up the heart and circulatory system we recommend a systematic, prudent exercise programme. And since the amount of blood pumped by the heart rises to its maximal at fairly low levels of exercise, we recommend that you never work at exercise intensities which you might describe as 'hard'; it's unnecessary, unproductive and could be dangerous. If you haven't exercised for a while, you may experience a certain amount of early discomfort. That's natural and will soon go away. We strongly recommend that you begin your exercise programme slowly and very gradually build your body to its potential over months and years. You didn't become unfit overnight and you shouldn't try to regain lost fitness in a few days.

The changes that will occur in your body as a result of a good exercise programme are several and have been well documented by exercise scientists. Some of the chief benefits of the training effect include: less fat, more muscle, better lungs, and of course a healthier heart and circulatory system.

41

CHAPTER 4

AN ANALYSIS
OF PHYSICAL FITNESS

It is probably an exaggeration to suggest that the initiation of an exercise programme will radically alter your life. However, it is fair to promise that most people who exercise will feel that it improves the quality of their life in some undefinable way. In this chapter we want to analyze critically this alteration in life's quality, to define its dimensions.

PHYSICAL FITNESS

Since 'physical fitness' is the most commonly heard term for that which is obtained when one exercises, the term clearly needs to be scrutinized in a book on exercise. What is physical fitness all about? Is physical fitness one, unitary, measurable construct? How does one go about developing and maintaining it? It is almost axiomatic that when an individual exercises, he or she expects to become physically fit. But what does that mean?

If we asked a series of experts to offer a precise definition of physical fitness we might hear a different definiton from each one. For us, physical fitness — at least in the context of this book — refers to the several human abilities needed to an adequate degree for the positive health of an individual[1]. Our definition includes an important reference to 'positive health'. We believe that attainment of physical fitness has a positive quality which transcends the familiar 'freedom from disease' concept. Physically fit individuals have not only maximized the capability of their body to withstand disease but they have also experienced a sense of awareness which we can only refer to as 'positive health'.

---

[1] Since this book has attempted to portray an 'exercise is good for everyone' theme, our definition here does not include a mention of the obvious implications of physical fitness in the readiness for motor/sport performance. This topic has been discussed by Burke (see references page 164).

And health refers to the whole body, especially the central nervous system upon which we rely for our conscious feeling of 'being alive'.

While there may be discrepencies among authorities in defining fitness, most could agree on what physical fitness is not! It is not a single unitary construct measured by one or even a few tests. Rather, a significant body of scientific literature, using the statistical tool of factor analysis, has firmly established that physical fitness consists of several abilities which we may call the components of physical fitness. The components most related to health are shown in Figure 4.1.

For the purpose of this discussion, we will consider physical fitness as consisting of five separate, fairly distinct abilities. Each is measured differently and, more importantly, each is developed by different types of training principles. A fuller understanding of these principles will permit better analysis of the goals for exercise.

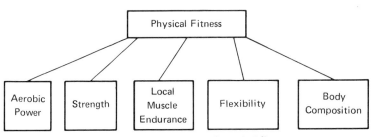

Fig. 4.1 The components of physical fitness

Aerobic power

Aerobic power is mentioned a great deal in this book. Obviously, we believe that this is a truly important human ability. Although the term aerobic power is preferred, the ability is sometimes called cardio-vascular or circulo-respiratory endurance, wind, stamina, being in shape, or just being fit. Several systems of the body are involved in the manifestation of this ability but it has particular significance because of its strong relationship with circulatory health.

In order to process great amounts of oxygen, the heart must be capable of pumping large quantities of blood. The rationale is widely accepted that a heart capable of pumping large quantities of blood per unit time (stroke volume) will have good healthy muscle.

Another factor in circulatory health is the efficiency of the blood vessels. You will remember that the circulatory system is a closed loop system of canals or tubes. The walls of the blood vessels are provided with smooth muscles which contract upon stimulation of the autonomic nervous system. Like all muscle, the smooth muscle in the walls of the blood vessels becomes more efficient with use. The blood vessels increase in elasticity and size; they also tend to increase in number. All of these alterations tend to be a net advantage in the battle against heart disease.

Still another characteristic consistent with improved aerobic power is improvement in the quality of the blood. As a result of aerobic exercise, you develop more blood. In addition, the oxygen-carrying elements, red blood cells and haemoglobin, develop more fully.

Aerobic power, as most human abilities, is powerfully influenced by heredity. Vassilis Klissouras of McGill University in Montreal has described a remarkable similarity in the aerobic power of identical twins in comparison with fraternal twins. He estimates that over ninety per cent of aerobic power is inherited.

Further substantiating the importance of genetic influence of aerobic power is the consistent finding that children are only capable of five to ten per cent improvement. However, because of the detrimental effect of sedentary life, average adults in western society are usually capable of fifteen to thirty per cent improvement. Far greater percentage improvements are possible in coronary patients. In one fascinating account, Doctors Terry Kavanagh and Roy Shephard of the University of Toronto described several middle-aged male heart attack victims who improved to the point where each was capable of participating in the Boston Marathon!

The test for aerobic power is the $\dot{V}O_2$ max test. This has been shown to be highly reproducible and seems to measure an important human ability, since it relates so well to circulatory efficiency. Unfortunately, the test requires expensive and sophisticated equipment, for example, a treadmill, bicycle ergometer, and oxygen/carbon dioxide analysis. It is therefore unlikely that most individuals will ever be directly tested for $\dot{V}O_2$ max.

For the analytical individual who wants to learn more about his or her capabilities, it is possible to obtain an accurate prediction of aerobic power by determining how far he or she can run in twelve minutes. Appropriate categories and approximate values for $\dot{V}O_2$ max in relation to the twelve-minute run score of a motivated individual are listed in chapter 10. It must be emphasized that the test should *never* be undertaken by anyone over the age of 35 who has not first consulted a doctor. And we recommend that these people be in an aerobic programme of the type described throughout this book for *at least six months* before undertaking such a vigorous test. On the other hand, for young fit people, the test is perfectly safe and should be given widely and often by physical education instructors as a means of motivating the young for the maintenance of this ability.

In his best-selling book, *Aerobics* (Bantam Books), Dr Kenneth

Cooper has created a list of exercises, each with a 'Cooper point' value. He has hypothesized that everyone should get at least thirty points for adequate aerobic fitness. He bases his theory on findings showing that nearly everyone who exercised at the thirty point level eventually was able to run 1½ miles in twelve minutes[2].

Cooper's point programme is very appealing for many, especially those who like a rigid, structured system. Although our experience with hundreds of healthy middle-aged adults is totally consistent with that of Dr Cooper, it may be that some individuals might prefer a less structured approach. We have found the following guidelines useful in establishing an aerobic training programme for healthy adults:

1 The primary activity should involve the large muscles of your body, i.e., those of the legs and arms.

2 The activity should be continuous and rhythmic for a period of several minutes.

3 The activity should involve an increase in heart rate and breathing rate, and usually some sweating. An exception to this rule is walking, where aerobic training benefits are possible but the time to obtain them is considerably longer (perhaps three to four times).

4 In examining the Borg scale of perceived exertion (see Table 5.4, page 67), you should not have to consider the exercise as being 'hard'. On the other hand, to obtain optimal benefits, neither should the exercise be considered 'light'. Aerobic exercise should be somewhere in between, i.e., between twelve and fourteen.

5 You should participate in each exercise session with a proper warm-up, stimulus period, and cool-down.

6 Three to four times per week is optimal.

7 Begin your programme with exercise of the type described for five to twenty minutes[3] per day. Gradually increase to a total of one to one and a half hours[3] of aerobic exercise per week (see chapter 5).

In closing, it may be noted that the best activities for achieving aerobic benefits are jogging, swimming, cycling, cross country skiing, and certain kinds of dancing. Sports such as basketball, soccer, and squash also develop the ability but require a physical structure which relatively few people possess.

Strength and local muscle endurance

The nature of muscle is such that when it is used it appears firm and usually grows in size based upon the intensity of the work performed.

[2]Which in turn usually signifies a 'healthy' aerobic power in the low forties.

[3]These values refer only to the 'aerobic' aspect of the programme. We also strongly recommend an approximately equal time spent in warm-up and cool-down. In chapter 5 we recommend the goal of three hours of exercise per week.

For women, the potential for increase in size is greatly reduced. The precise biochemical stimulus is unknown, but the muscle cell responds to prolonged periods of tension by 1) an increase in the thickness of the cell wall; 2) an increase in the fluid content of the cell; and 3) usually an increase in the vascularity (number of blood vessels) of the cell. These physiological alterations can be summarized by a descriptive term called hypertrophy, i.e., the muscle gets larger in size. Whatever the biochemical processes are, it helps to have testosterone, the male sex hormone, available. Women are at a decided disadvantage in increasing the size of muscle because of a relative lack of this hormone.

Unfortunately, for many in our modern technological society a reverse of muscle build-up is also possible. Muscles that are not used look flabby and are known to decrease in size.

From the above it follows that the muscle mass of the body is malleable. Although we all have some indefinable hereditary limitation on size and strength, it is most certainly true that for most individuals a great deal of improvement is possible. In our personal experience with many young men and women, we have found it not at all uncommon to see forty to sixty per cent improvement in the strength of certain muscle groups after just twelve weeks of training of the type which we will be describing here and in chapter 6.

Dr Jack Wilmore, when he was doing research at the University of California-Davis, found that women improved at a rate similar to men in most muscle groups as a result of a standard isotonic weight training programme. You can get extra stength if you want it!

Strength

Muscle strength may be defined as the ability of the muscle or muscle group to apply force with one maximal contraction. Thus, an individual who can curl fifty pounds has more muscle strength of the biceps than someone who can curl thirty pounds. As hinted earlier, strong people usually have bigger muscles than weaker ones. There are, however, some individuals who may be termed 'wiry', who do not look strong but have the ability to apply a great amount of force because of favourable leverage, i.e., their bones are arranged favourably for application of strength. Another possible reason for the strength of some who 'don't look it' may be related to the nervous input to their muscles. The muscles receive excitatory and inhibitory nervous input. Inhibitory nervous input seems to be a mechanism to prevent the muscle from literally pulling itself away from the bone. Some individuals may be able to reduce the inhibitory input and thus exert more force for a given amount of muscle.

In order to discuss strength training fully, we need to analyze such terms as isotonics, isometrics, isokinetics, concentric and eccentric contractions. We will do that in chapter 6. In this chapter we will try to summarize strength development in lifting a freely moving weight through a range of motion (barbells).

Thanks in part to the original research of Dr Richard Berger of Temple University, the following simple guidelines should be followed for optimal strength development:

1 Every contraction should be made through the full range of motion. Far from the myth that weight training will cause 'muscle boundness', there is an abundance of research showing that flexibility will be improved if this is done.

2 Almost any systematic overload (increased tension) procedure will result in improved muscle strength. Based primarily on the work of Berger, the most efficient method is probably for the individual to work at a resistance equal to or greater than his or her 6RM (maximal repetitions). This means that the weight lifted should be so heavy that the individual is incapable of lifting it more than six times consecutively.

3 Each of these 2 to 6RM sessions is a set. Three to four sets should be done each training day. Allow five to ten minutes between sets for a given muscle group.

4 As the individual becomes able to lift a given resistance more than six times, increase the resistance 5 to 7 lbs for men: 2½ to 5 lbs for a women.

5 Make your training as nearly identical to a desired sport skill as possible (if there is one).

6 A corollary to point 5 is to emphasize that you continue to practise a given motor skill during the strength-training period. For example, if you are a golfer, continue to play golf during the period of strength improvement.

7 Train a given set of muscles on an every-other-day basis. For example, you may wish to work on the arms and chest muscles on Monday, Wednesday, Friday, the legs and abdominal muscles on Tuesday, Thursday, Saturday. It may be added that only the most ardent of weight trainers work on an every-day basis. We suggest that you choose your goals and work one to three days per week.

Perhaps the prime (health-related) benefit of extra strength is related to bodily appearance. A given weight of muscle takes up less space than fat — you lose inches. The fat, bulging waistline of many individuals is not favoured by our society.

Strength improvement has other positive health advantages. Improvement in muscle strength and tone is almost always accompanied by a heightened sense of muscular awareness. Physiologists have described several types of receptors in skeletal muscles, each providing the individual with the 'sixth sense' of touch and position in space. Almost everyone who 'tones up' describes a wonderful new feeling of being alive, which is difficult to quantify but nonetheless real.

Other health-related aspects are also possible. We should not under-estimate the advantages of strength in providing proper posture. Several physicians have cited the negative effects on internal organs from poor posture which often results from weak muscles. Weak abdominal muscles can clearly lead to lower back pain — the curse of many for several decades of their life.

Local muscle endurance

Local muscle endurance (LME) refers to the ability of a muscle or group of muscles in a specific part of the body to work effectively over a period of time. With the exception of the degree of tension employed, all of the principles of strength training apply in the development of LME. In strength training, the individual applies such great force (muscle tension) that contractions can only be carried on for a short period of time, i.e. high resistance, low repetitions. In contrast, LME may be improved with lower levels of tension spread over longer periods of time, i.e. low resistance, high repetitions. In this regard special equip-ment is not needed for the development of LME. The body is used as the resistance to be moved in a wide variety of calisthenic exercises, illustrated in chapters 5 and 7. For example, to do a series of bent knee sit-ups is to be working on the development of LME.

Associated with development of muscle endurance is the develop-ment of muscle tone. That is, muscles which are regularly contracted tend to become firm and taut, as opposed to the flabby muscle of the non-exerciser. To develop LME is to 'firm up'.

Flexibility

Flexibility refers to the range of possible movements about a joint or sequence of joints. Flexibility is affected by 1) the degree of stretch and position of attachment of connective tissue such as ligaments and tendons, 2) the shape and size of the muscles and 3) the shape, size, and arrangement of bones.

As might be expected, flexibility is most certainly affected by heredity. In general, women have greater flexibility than men for several reasons. Their lesser degree of musculature permits a freer movement at the joints. Possibly more important is the female hormone, relaxin, which is available to permit the stretching of the pelvis during childbirth, but also provides for the greater stretch of connective tissue, for example, ligaments which attach bones to each other and tendons which attach muscles to bone.

Flexibility exercises are similar to those that promote local muscle endurance and muscle tone. Although the effect of such exercise is difficult to assess objectively, most individuals who consciously improve their flexibility do so with a feeling of overall bodily well-being.

According to Greg Bostwick of the Department of Drama at Ithaca College, it is widely accepted in drama circles that certain exercises are able to instil in actors a new-found feeling of self-confidence. Flexibility exercises (such as Yoga) seem to create in the individual a perceived 'energy flow' streaming outward from the centre of the body. The ability to project onself is enhanced. Another benefit may be a heightened sensitivity to stimuli, clearly important for an actor.

In the short run, exercises may help the individual to deal with physical stress, for example going on stage. Tight muscles can impair creativity. A taut, toned, flexible body can make it easier to feel that 'I can handle it'.

Other benefits may also accrue to those who develop flexibility. As we meet people in our daily life, we constantly give signs and cues to them about who and what we are. From the recently emerging science of body language we know that individuals with flexible, toned bodies are better able to project an image of self-confidence.

Realists — scientists interested in measurement — might criticize such speculation. They might argue that such feelings as 'self-confidence' or 'I can handle it' are impossible to measure and therefore it is wrong to attribute such benefits as these to the effects of exercise. To these individuals it is argued that we are pathetically ignorant concerning the workings of the central nervous system. The 'feelings' expressed by almost everyone who regularly participates in Yoga, dance or similar activities should not be dismissed by physiologists simply because we cannot measure them[4]. The eminent cell biologist, Lewis Thomas, tells us:

'The only solid piece of scientific truth about which I feel totally confident is that we are profoundly ignorant about nature. Indeed, I regard this as the major discovery of the past hundred years of biology . . . It is this sudden confrontation with the depth and scope of ignorance that represents the most significant contribution of twentieth century science to the human intellect.'

Body composition

To many, body composition is the most important of the components of physical fitness. Women consistently rank weight control as the most significant reason for exercise. In western society, leanness is glorified. Everyone, or so it sometimes seems, is worried about his or her body.

---

[4]The exciting new results from the 'Endorphin' research may provide tangible reasons for self confidence, etc., resulting from stretching and other Yoga-type exercise.

Body composition is perhaps the easiest of the components of physical fitness to recognize. But there are several ways of assessing the external dimensions of your body. Height is one criterion for evaluating the body. Unfortunately, we cannot do a thing about our height and so there is little point in worrying about it. Another measure is body type. For this discussion, body type refers to the arrangement and relative size of bones, along with the relative predisposition to musculature and fat deposit. We can be rated along three categories — endomorphic, mesomorphic and ectomorphic (see Figure 4.2). Most of us have a combination of traits in each category. The endomorph has short, thick bones with a tendency to extra fat in the abdominal area. The ectomorph is usually low in fat and muscle, with long thin bones. Finally, the mesomorph is muscular with wide shoulders and narrow hips. Your underlying bony structure cannot be altered. However, since fat and muscle are definitely affected by diet and exercise, it is possible, to some extent, to alter the appearance of your basic body type.

The aspect of body type which undergoes the greatest alteration thoughout your lifetime is weight (see Table 4.1). In analysis of body weight, it is useful to divide arbitrarily the body into non-fat (lean) and

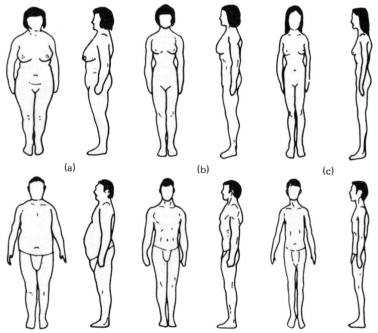

(a) (b) (c)

Fig. 4.2 Three extreme body types; (a) endomorph, (b) mesomorph, (c) ectomorph

fat compartments. As with most aspects of your body, your fat stores are partially affected by heredity. Males in general have less fat than females. The percentage of fat distribution ranges from twelve to twenty-four per cent in males and nineteen to thirty per cent in females. Some athletes may be found with fat distribution below this range but in non-athletes it is usually a sign of being thin. Individuals found above this range are considered to be approaching obesity.

The reason the average male has less fat than the average female is clear. Males have the sex hormone testosterone which is of benefit in making muscle. Females have only minute amounts of the hormone, and therefore have a greater tendency to go to fat[5].

Exercise can help in your battle against undesired fat weight in several ways. A quick review of Appendix B will reveal calorie expenditure of varying types of exercise. If all other factors are held constant, you can expect to lose about one pound of fat per month from the type of exercise programme to be described in the next chapter.

Next, exercise can help by reducing your appetite. That's right! You eat more when you do not exercise than when you do — up to a point. For centuries, farmers have known that they can fatten up their hogs and cattle by penning them — denying them exercise.

Strength and toning exercises can help by building and firming muscle. Unused, flabby muscles look like more flabby fat. If you build muscle while holding your weight constant, you have to be losing fat. You also have to be losing inches, since muscle takes up a lot less space than fat. And a firm, toned muscle is another source of calorie expenditure — every little bit helps!

SUMMARY

In this chapter we have attempted to define the boundaries of the health-related aspects of physical fitness. A better understanding of the implications of each of the components of physical fitness may help lead you to a wiser selection of exercise goals. We hope that you are now ready for a fuller analysis of systematic, prudent exercise in the chapters which follow.

---

[5] As we intimated in chapter 2, these greater fat reserves are clearly needed to ensure adequate energy for both the mother and the foetus in times of scarcity, to improve survival chances.

Table 4.1 Weight tables for men and women (weight in pounds according to frame — in indoor clothing)

Desirable Weights for Men, Ages 25 and over

Height (with shoes on) 1-in. heels		Small frame	Medium frame	Large frame
ft.	in.			
5	2	112–120	118–129	126–141
5	3	115–123	121–133	129–144
5	4	118–126	124–136	132–148
5	5	121–129	127–139	135–152
5	6	124–133	130–143	138–158
5	7	128–137	134–147	142–161
5	8	132–141	138–152	147–166
5	9	136–145	142–156	151–170
5	10	140–150	146–160	155–174
5	11	144–154	150–165	159–179
6	0	148–158	154–170	164–184
6	1	152–162	158–175	168–189
6	2	156–167	162–180	173–194
6	3	160–171	167–185	178–199
6	4	164–175	172–190	182–204

Desirable Weights for Women, Ages 25 and over

Height (with shoes on) 1-in. heels ft.	in.	Small frame	Medium frame	Large frame
4	10	92– 98	96–107	104–119
4	11	94–101	98–110	106–119
5	0	96–104	101–113	109–125
5	1	99–107	104–116	112–128
5	2	102–110	107–119	115–131
5	3	105–113	110–122	118–134
5	4	108–116	113–126	121–138
5	5	111–119	116–130	125–142
5	6	114–123	120–135	129–146
5	7	118–127	124–139	133–150
5	8	112–131	128–143	137–154
5	9	126–135	132–147	141–158
5	10	130–140	136–151	145–163
5	11	134–144	140–155	149–168
6	0	138–148	144–159	153–173

For girls between 18 and 25, subtract 1 lb. for each year under 25.

CHAPTER 5

EXERCISE: WHAT, WHERE AND HOW

At this point you are probably convinced that exercise is a good idea but you have many questions. How should I begin? What is the best type of exercise programme for me? How much exercise is enough? How hard should I work? How do I progress? This chapter is designed to answer all of these questions and others that may be of interest to anyone embarking on an exercise programme.

GOALS

Perhaps the first step in developing a prudent exercise programme is to establish a set of goals (see Table 5.1). Why do you want to exercise? In the last chapter we outlined the components of physical fitness, attempting to make a case that aerobic power is of the highest importance for most people. However, your own first priority might be fat loss. Both aerobic power and fat loss are accomplished by the type of exercise programme outlined here.

Table 5.1 Possible goals for an exercise programme

Goal	Check
Aerobic (cardio-vascular)	( )
Anaerobic (all-out work) – *for athletes*	( )
Strength (size of muscle)	( )
Local muscle endurance (muscle tone)	( )
Flexibility (range of motion)	( )
Fat loss	( )
Self confidence	( )
Positive sense of 'being alive'	( )

Muscle tone and flexibility may be your preferred goals. There is an almost mystical feeling of overall bodily well-being associated with a toned, flexible body. Both muscle tone and flexibility may be improved by the type of exercise programme which we are going to recommend. However, other forms of exercise may also be important. Yoga has a particular appeal for many and you may wish to explore this type of exercise.

If strength and muscle enlargement rank high, you will want to read chapter 6 in which we discuss the best and most efficient techniques for increasing the size and strength of muscle.

Little will be said in this book about the development of the anaerobic potential of the body. Our belief is that all-out, sprint type work is a matter strictly for athletes. For health-related fitness, you just do not need anaerobic power. There is simply no reason for all-out bursts of work lasting fifteen seconds to a few minutes. Unfortunately, many people think that you have to have a burst of speed or have to be sweating heavily and working very hard to achieve fitness. This is not true. The best forms of exercise, to achieve the goals of fitness which we believe are most important, involve work well within your limits — not at all near to your maximum potential.

There are less objective, but nonetheless real, goals of exercise, such as self-confidence and improved self-image. Assuming that you are one of those individuals who have not been doing much for several years, exercise of the type to be proposed cannot help but brighten your outlook on life — and almost immediately.

GETTING STARTED

You have decided that aerobic exercise is for you. What is your first step? We cannot emphasize the answer to this question too strongly. If you are over thirty-five years of age consult your doctor. He or she knows what is best for your health. It would be foolish to follow the recommendation of a book — the authors of which know nothing about you — without consulting the person who knows most about your body. Only your doctor is in a position to diagnose the several conditions which either preclude physical exercise or call for greater caution (see Appendix D). The overwhelming majority of doctors want to prevent disease just as much as you do. While doctors do not always have a great deal of knowledge about exercise, they almost universally recommend prudent exercise. And in the unlikely event that a doctor tells you *not* to exercise, do not go out and exercise — get a second opinion. After a good check-up and a talk with your doctor, you will be ready to start. If you are planning to combine exercise with a diet to lose weight, be sure to tell your doctor.

For individuals of thirty-five or less, it is less important to see a doctor, but nonetheless a prudent act. The value of a yearly physical check-up is not to be minimized. The curious reality is that most of us provide better maintenance for our house, garden, and car than we do for our body.

JOGGING IS BEST

Of the forms of exercise available to improve aerobic power and to help with fat control, jogging undoubtedly has the most advantages. Unlike other forms of exercise, jogging is not weather dependent. Except on a very few days each year, you can go out and run. Sport centres are growing up all over Great Britain. Many have running programmes and times of the day when you can go for a run.

Swimming, cycling, and cross-country skiing are excellent, but each is dependent on something special. Swimming depends upon good weather or an indoor pool (with hundreds of bathers in your way). Cycling requires an expensive bicycle, and is somewhat unsafe in many cities. Cycling is also far more enjoyable with a less hilly topography than that found in parts of the British Isles.

Perhaps the best form of exercise of all is cross-country skiing, demanding the continuous use of nearly every muscle in the body. However, it obviously requires a great deal more snow than is common in many countries.

In summary, then, we are presenting jogging as the cheapest, most efficient and accessible form of exercise for most people.

Choosing a running shoe

One of the first steps in beginning a running programme is to purchase a good pair of shoes. Orthopaedic problems are perhaps the most common reason for individuals dropping out of running programmes. Swollen ankles and knees are not uncommon. And even more prevalent is the dreaded shin splint. In this injury, the individual feels sharp pains in the front of the lower leg with even mild exertion. The condition makes running difficult, if not impossible. Many, if not most, orthopaedic problems could have been avoided with proper precautions. Good shoes are an important first step in the prevention of the so called 'overuse' injury. You should go to a reputable footwear store — one where the sales people have the time to talk to you. Tell them that you want to purchase a running shoe. If they begin by telling you that a tennis shoe is just as good, you are in the wrong shop.

Several factors should influence your decision about a running shoe. The shoe should be able to provide cushioning for the ball of the foot. It should have a firm arch support, as well as enough flexibility to provide for easy push-off. The foot should be measured while you are in the standing position, and in the late afternoon or early evening, since the feet swell during the day. This point is particularly critical for women because of the cyclical fluid shifts of their body.

Examine your running shoe in comparison with the fully labelled shoe in Figure 5.1. The heel counter should fit snugly, yet not be so stiff as to cause limitation. The vamp should be wide enough for the fore-foot. Finally, the toe box should permit free movement of the toes without pressure.

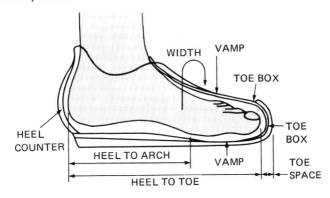

Fig. 5.1 The running shoe labelled

Other precautions

Many beginning runners run on their toes. This is clearly wrong and can lead to orthopaedic problems. Running is a heel and toe movement. Land on your heel and push off from your toe. You may have to con-centrate on this point for a while, but very soon it will become second nature for you.

Some people have a gait in which their toes point out at a forty-five degree angle at each foot strike. Force yourself to point your toes as nearly directly forward as possible. This may be difficult for some, but studies have shown a higher incidence of shin splints in runners who 'toe out'.

The type of surface on which you run is also important. Grass and dirt paths are the best. Try to stay off hard roads or surfaces built over hard concrete. The podiatrist, Donald Maron, also recommends his personal technique for lacing a shoe (Figure 5.2). Try it and we believe you will notice a difference.

Do not run in the same direction every day. If you run inside, try to run clockwise half of the time and vice versa. When you always run in the same direction, the leg muscles responsible for the inside leg may develop differently from the outside leg. The compensation needed during straight running may result in undue stress on one of the legs, leading to problems like swelling of the knee or ankle. The stress on the supporting structures — tendons, bones, and ligaments — of the legs caused by running should not be minimized. In a mile run, there may be up to one thousand foot strikes, each at a force of three to six times your body weight.

At each foot strike there is normally a slight pronation or turning inward of the foot. If you have a small abnormality in the arrangement of the structures of the foot, there can result an abnormally long period of pronation. The resulting twisting motion, as the body attempts to get balanced, may cause damage when repeated thousands of times.

If you have attempted to comply with the earlier suggestions and yet still experience pain of an orthopaedic nature, then be sure to consult an orthopaedic surgeon or a podiatrist. Often doctors specializing in sports medicine can fit you with an 'orthotic'. This shoe insert is designed to tell your foot bones 'where to go'. The device assists the foot in landing flat, resulting in a greater balance of the body at foot strike.

Although we know, and want you to know, that there is the possibility of problems of the type just described with running, we believe that the benefits far outweigh the risks. If you proceed *slowly* and comply with all of our suggestions, the chances are that you will not be affected by these problems.

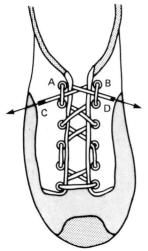

Fig. 5.2 Maron lacing technique

1. Lift up lace A, pull lace C under lace A
2. Lift up lace B, pull lace D under lace B
3. Pull tight in direction of arrows
4. Tie in usual manner

YOUR INDIVIDUAL EXERCISE PROGRAMME

For you to achieve your goals of exercise most efficiently, each of the following considerations has importance: warm-up, stimulus, duration, intensity, frequency, progression and cool-down.

Warm-up

It is wise to spend ten to fifteen minutes warming up. The reasons are several. You should gradually prepare the heart and other structures of the body for the upcoming training stimulus. During warm-up the body can begin to get the blood flowing to the large muscles, especially in the legs. Furthermore, the warmed muscle is better able to use the oxygen being sent in the blood stream. There is less need to make lactic acid.

Warm-up also has implications for injury prevention. Gradual stretching of the muscles, ligaments, and tendons may result in fewer strains, sprains, and pulls.

It is important to contract as many muscles as possible. Proceed gradually from easy exercises to more difficult ones. In this way, you can be toning as many muscles as possible while stretching the joints, thus improving flexibility.

We have found that, with people of all ages, music is a great addition to an exercise programme, especially during this warm-up phase. There is a mysterious (but nonetheless real) symbiotic relationship between the rhythmic contraction of your muscles and music. Music and exercise makes you feel good!

As you pick exercises from Figure 5.3, several considerations are pertinent. Begin slowly with relatively easy exercises. Choose a variety of exercises so that as many muscles are contracted as possible. Perhaps you may wish to alternate your exercises on different days. On the first day, begin with a few repetitions — five to ten — of each exercise chosen. As you proceed with your programme regularly add to the number of repetitions.

Perhaps the most important of the exercises are ones which work to tone and strengthen the abdominal muscles. Be sure to do some bent-knee sit-ups every training day. Many people go through most of their life with low back pain — and this could have been avoided by keeping their abdominal muscles strong. Begin with five to ten good, slow bent-knee sit-ups (see also chapter 6). For the execution of this movement see abdominal strengthener 1 page 87.

Static stretching

The well-known physiologist, Herbert de Vries, of the University of Southern California has developed an important theory which must be considered in the analysis of a good running programme. He notes that exercise can sometimes cause a localized lack of blood supply. This may be particularly true when the individual has not run for a long time or in those individuals who do a great deal of running (five to fifteen miles) at a given time. A lack of blood supply to the leg muscle may result in pain, which may in turn cause a heightening of muscle contraction, provoking an even greater contraction. Thus he believes that the resulting muscle spasm may be one of the causes of the more severe pain of shin splints.

His recommendations are simple. In order to get the muscle out of contraction, you stretch it for a period of time. A few years ago, de Vries recommended some static stretches for our adult fitness programme. Since these stretches have been incorporated into the programme, a decline in the incidence of orthopaedic problems has been noted. So, we strongly recommend that you do each of the four static stretches described and illustrated in Figure 5.3 immediately after your warm-up, and again, following your cool-down walk. (Other excellent exercises are described in chapter 7.)

Stimulus period

This is, of course, the most important aspect of each day's exercise programme. Following the research of the great Swedish physiologist, Per Olof Astrand, we strongly recommend interval training.

Interval training refers to a training programme in which you intersperse work (runs during the stimulus period) with regular rest (walking) intervals. You are using the same number of calories, yet breaking up the runs. This has both psychological and physiological advantages. You tell yourself — at least for the first few days — that 'I can put up with anything for a few minutes'. The rests permit you to do a lot more total work and may be a better positive stimulus for the muscles (particularly the heart muscle) than a continuous run. It is not true that exercise has to cause pain to give benefit. Anything this easy *can* be good. Based upon experience with hundreds of exercisers of all ages, we strongly encourage beginners to initiate their programme with interval training.

Duration and intensity

How far do I go? How fast do I go? The answer to these questions are the keys to a safe, sound exercise programme. In order to answer them intelligently, you first need to classify yourself in one of the categories of Table 5.2. (It is assumed that if you are over thirty-five years you will have seen your doctor first.)

Several conclusions can be drawn from Table 5.2. You can see that the most important factors in assigning your first day's exercise are your recent activity patterns, your age, your sex, your smoking habits, and your (fat) weight. Considering these factors, you can make an edu-

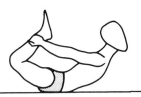
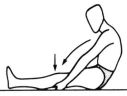

Thigh stretch. In a prone position, reach back with both hands and clasp the ankles. Slowly lift the legs up and off the ground forming a cradle position. Hold in the stretched position for 10 to 12 seconds, relax and repeat.

Hamstring stretch. In a sitting position with the knees flat against the floor, slowly move the upper body toward the knees. Hold in the stretched position for 10 to 12 seconds, relax and repeat.

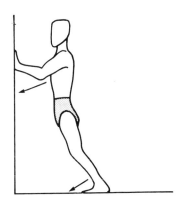

Heel cord stretch. With the arms outstretched, the hands against the wall and the heels flat on the floor, the elbows are bent to allow the body to gradually lean forward. This stretch should be held for 10 to 12 counts and repeated several times.

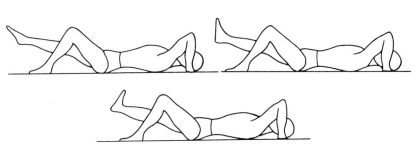

This involves three stages with each held for 7 seconds. Begin in a supine position with one leg flexed and the other extended and off the floor. Stage one involves full ankle plantar flexion; two is a mid-range hold; and three is full dorsi-flexion. Move through all stages and repeat with the other leg. Three complete sets are recommended for each leg.

Fig. 5.3 Static stretches

61

Table 5.2 Beginning an exercise programme

Which set of phrases in the CATEGORY column best descibes you? Make a check in the ( ). CATEGORY	INTENSITY (Speed during the run. The walk may be any speed which is comfort-able).	DURATION (Intervals of work and rest e.g., 3—1 means run three minutes then walk one minute).
( ) Under 25 years of age, plenty of recent exercise*, a male	D	3—1, 3—1 3—1, 3—1
( ) Under 25 years of age, plenty of recent exercise*, a female	E	3—1, 3—1 3—1, 3—1
( ) Under 25 years of age, little or no recent exercise, a male	E	2—1, 2—1 2—1, 2—1
( ) Under 25 years of age, little or no recent exercise, a female	F	2—1, 2—1 2—1, 2—1
( ) Under 25 years of age, little or no recent exercise, a male and little overweight** or a smoker	F	2—1, 2—1 2—1
( ) Under 25 years of age, little or no recent exercise, a female and overweight** or a smoker	G	2—1, 2—1 2—1
( ) Under 25 years of age, little or no recent exercise, an over-weight** male smoker	G	1—1, 1—1 1—1, 1—1 1—1
( ) Under 25 years of age, little or no recent exercise, an over-weight female smoker	H	1—1, 1—1 1—1, 1—1 1—1
( ) 25 to 35 years of age, plenty of recent exercise, a male	E	2—1, 2—1 2—1, 2—1
( ) 25 to 35 years of age, plenty of recent exercise, a female	F	2—1, 2—1 2—1, 2—1
( ) 25 to 35 years of age, little or no recent exercise, a male	F	2—1, 2—1 2—1
( ) 25 to 35 years of age, little or no recent exercise, a female	G	2—1, 2—1 2—1

	CATEGORY	INTENSITY	DURATION
( )	25 to 35 years of age, little or no recent exercise, a male and over-weight or a smoker	G	1–1, 1–1 1–1, 1–1 1–1
( )	25 to 35 years of age, little or no recent exercise, a female and little overweight** or a smoker	H	1–1, 1–1 1–1, 1–1
( )	25 to 35 years of age, little or no recent exercise, an overweight** male smoker	H	1–1, 1–1 1–1, 1–1
( )	25 to 35 years of age, little or no recent exercise, an overweight** female smoker	I	1–1, 1–1 1–1, 1–1
( )	36 to 49**, plenty of recent exercise, a male	F	2–1, 2–1 2–1
( )	36 to 49**, plenty of recent exercise, a female	G	2–1, 2–1 2–1
( )	36 to 49**, little or no recent exercise, a male	G	1 1/2–1, 1 1/2–1, 1 1/2–1
( )	36 to 49**, little or no recent exercise, a female	H	1 1/2–1, 1 1/2–1 1 1/2–1
( )	36 to 49**, little or no recent exercise, a male and either overweight*** or a smoker	G	1–1, 1–1 1–1, 1–1
( )	36 to 49**, little or no recent exercise, a female and either overweight*** or a smoker	H	1–1, 1–1 1–1, 1–1
( )	36 to 49**, little or no recent exercise, an overweight*** male smoker	G	1/2–1, 1/2–1 1/2–1 1/2–1
( )	36 to 49**, little or no recent exercise, an overweight***female smoker	H	1/2–1, 1/2–1 1/2–1
( )	Age 50** or greater, plenty of recent exercise, a male	G	2–1, 2–1 2–1

CATEGORY		INTENSITY	DURATION
( )	Age 50** or greater, plenty of recent exercise, a female	H	2—1, 2—1 2—1
( )	Age 50** or greater, little or no recent exercise, a male	H	1—2, 1—2 1—2
( )	Age 50** or greater, little or no recent exercise, a female	I	1—2, 1—2 1—2
( )	Age 50** or greater, little or no recent exercise, a male and either overweight*** or a smoker	I	1/2—2, 1/2—2, 1/2—2 1/2—2
( )	Age 50** or greater, little or no recent exercise, an overweight female	I	1/2—2, 1/2—2 1/2—2 1/2—2
( )	Age 50** or greater, little or no recent exercise, an overweight male smoker	I	1/2—2, 1/2—2 1/2—2
( )	Age 50** or greater, little or no recent exercise, an overweight female smoker	I	1/2—2, 1/2—2 1/2—2

*Plenty of recent exercise implies that you have been doing aerobic exercise for at least ½ hour, 2—3 times a week for the last several months. Of course, if the exercise has been running, there is no need for this table. Continue what you've been doing.

**Overweight according to the criteria described in Appendix A or Table 1, Chapter 4.

*** The prescription of intensity and duration assumes that no other contraindications to exercise are present. These may be assessed in a good physical examination by a physician who realizes that you wish to become involved in an exercise programme.

cated guess as to what should be your first day's training stimulus. Some might find this early training too easy. But we hasten to state that you have become de-conditioned over several years, and you should not try to regain your reduced aerobic power in a few days!

To use Table 5.2, simply find the phrase, or phrases, which is most appropriate for you. Then, during the stimulus phase of your first day's training session, make the number of runs shown. For the speed, you will have to use Table 5.3. This provides the appropriate lap time, i.e. the time which you should take for *one* continuous lap, for several different marked distances. If you do not have a track or a gym to run round, you could take your car and mark off a set distance over a flat street in your area. With a little simple maths you could then arrive at the right time needed to achieve the correct speed.

Let me describe the nature of a given run for certain speeds. Intensities J–L are either very fast *walks* or very, very slow runs. H and I are slow runs – at first you almost have to force yourself to run so slowly. Intensities G and up are ever-increasing running speeds – you really need to measure off a distance to get these accurately. It is very interesting that, after a while most people are able to call upon their body to match these various speeds without a watch. We seem to have a biological clock for running speeds, but it needs a little practice.

We will now look at an example of the use of Table 5.2. If we have a forty-year-old housewife who has done little exercise in recent years (and has a go-ahead from her doctor), what should be her stimulus period during her first training session? This woman works round the house and a little in the garden, but that is all. She does not smoke but, in consulting Table 4.1 (page 52), she concludes that she is overweight. In her case, Table 5.2 indicates that she should run for a minute and walk for a minute, and continue the process for a total of four sets of run/walks. Further, she will find, on consulting Table 5.3, that she should run at an intensity of 5.3 mph, or at a very slow run.

When you have done your first day's exercise, you should evaluate yourself. We will look at two ways of doing this: perceived exertion and heart rate.

Perceived exertion
After your last run, simply ask yourself how you feel, according to the chart in Table 5.4. Gunnar Borg, of the University of Stockholm, developed this chart in the mid-sixties. We have found it an extremely valuable tool.

We saw in chapter 4 that the measure of aerobic power is the VO_2 max. Furthermore, in chapter 3 you learned that your stroke volume – the amount of blood pumped by your heart with each beat – is just about at its maximum at 65–70 per cent of $\dot{V}O_2$ max. We have

Table 5.3 Conversion of exercise intensities to calories expended per minute. (1)

Running/Walking

Intensity	⅛ mi track Time/lap (Sec)	¼ mi track Time/lap (Sec) (2)	1 mi track (Min: Sec)	26 Laps/ mi Track Time/Lap .5 (Sec)	Full Sized Basketball Court 18.75 Laps–mi. Time–Lap .5 Sec.	Km per Hour	Miles per Hour	Kcal (3) Per Min Expended During Exercise (4) nearest .5	
								Walk	Run
A	45	90	6:00	14.0	19.0	16.1	10.0		20
B	50	100	6:40	15.0	21.5	14.49	9.0		18
C	55	110	7:20	17.0	23.5	13.19	8.19		16
D	60	120	8:00	18.5	25.5	12.07	7.50		15
E	65	130	8:40	20.0	28.0	11.14	6.92		14
F	70	140	9:20	21.5	30.0	10.35	6.43		13
G	75	150	10:00	23.0	32.0	9.66	6.00		12.5
H	80	160	10:40	24.5	34.0	9.05	5.62		12
I	85	170	11:20	26.0	36.5	8.53	5.30		11
J	90*	180*	12:00*	27.5*	38.5*	8.05*	5.00*		11
K	95	190	12:40	29.5	40.5	7.62	4.73	8.5	10.5
L	100	200	13:20	30.0	42.5	7.25	4.50	8.0	10
M	105	210	14:00	32.5	45.0	6.90	4.29	7.5	9.5
N	110	220	14:40	34.0	47.0	6.58	4.09	6.5	9.0

(1) Values are accurate to approximately ± 10%

(2) For equivalent times on a 400 meter track, subtract 1 second from exercise intensities A through 0; subtract 2 seconds for exercise intensities P and Q; subtract 3 seconds for exercise intensity R.

(3) Assume a 70kg individual.

(4) At intensities greater than 50% of VO_2 max., the total calories cost is substantially greater (perhaps 20–40 %) due to anaerobic involvement, its inefficiency and the subsequent repayment in O_2 Debt. Evidence has been offered that the VO_2 max. of an individual may also affect the total calories expended at a given work level.

Table 5.4 The (RPE) scale for ratings of perceived exertion (Borg, 1971).

6	
7	Very, very light
8	
9	Very light
10	
11	Fairly light
12	
13	Somewhat hard
14	
15	Hard
16	
17	Very hard
18	
19	Very, very hard
20	

"Your goal is to rate your feelings which are caused by the work and not the work itself. These feelings should be general, that is about the body as a whole. We will not ask you to specify the feeling but to select a number which most accurately corresponds to your perception of your total body feeling. Keep in mind that there are no right or wrong numbers. Use any number you think is appropriate." (Noble, et al., 1973).

found through a great deal of research — some done at Leeds Polytechnic — that most individuals who say that they are at 12–14 are safely working at 70–75 per cent of VO_2 max level. And that is as hard as you have to work. If your response is 'hard' (15) perhaps you should slow up on the next day's exercise. Those who say 11 or less need more work to get enough results. If you say 16 or 17, be *sure* to slow up and work less.

This method is not as subjective as it might appear. Most people have the ability to know how close they are to their maximum. It is probably an inherited ability going back to the time when some hunts took days. Then, the efficient runners got their prey; the inefficient ones died out.

There is another way of testing that you are working at the desired training stimulus (70–75 per cent of $\dot{V}O_2$ max). Are you able to talk or carry on a conversation with a fellow runner? If not, slow up!

Heart rate
The most commonly employed check that you are running at the desired

training intensity is the use of heart rate (HR). Many experts would recommend that you work at an HR of seventy-five to eighty-five per cent of your maximum heart rate. Of course the problem is that it takes a very difficult test — which must be supervised by a doctor — to find your maximum heart rate. But we can give you an approximation — your HR max is equal to about 220 minus your age. For example, John is thirty years old. His predicted HR max is therefore 220 - 30 = 190. Since everyone should be working at between seventy-five and eighty-five per cent of HR max[1], his desired HR at the end of exercise should be between 143 and 162.

We always teach our runners to take their HR at the wrist. After exercise, it is quite easy to determine by putting your two forefingers next to the bone on the thumb side of your wrist. Count for ten seconds and multiply by six to get HR. John, in the example above, should have a post-run ten-second HR of between twenty-four and twenty-seven. Take your HR as near to the end of the last run as possible.

Heart rate and perceived exertion compared as measures of exercise intensity

The basis of a good, individualized exercise programme is to be working at your most efficient level of work — about seventy to seventy-five per cent of $\dot{V}O_2$ max. This means that a typical thirty-year-old should be working at a perceived exertion of 'somewhat hard' (12–14), or an HR of between 143 and 162. In practice we have found that these values work well together. When one is high the other is usually high, and so on. When one is too high, we would normally recommend caution. However, there are two instances where these two measures of intensity seem to vary. Many times, women have much higher heart rates than their perceived exertion would suggest. If a woman's HR is consistently at 180 or so and she feels that the work is 13 or less, this is a good work load for that woman. The opposite sometimes happens with smokers. One of the many prices they seem to have to pay for their smoking is an abnormally high perceived exertion for a given HR level. In the case of smokers, we are inclined to place more faith in HR as a measure of intensity.

Frequency

Make an attempt to plan your life so that you can participate in an exercise programme of the type described at least three days per week. We would recommend that you begin a thirty-minute programme based on a mix of stretching, running, walking, and cool-down exercises. Using

---

[1] This is approximately equal to our seventy-five per cent of $\dot{V}O_2$ max criterion for safe, effective exercise.

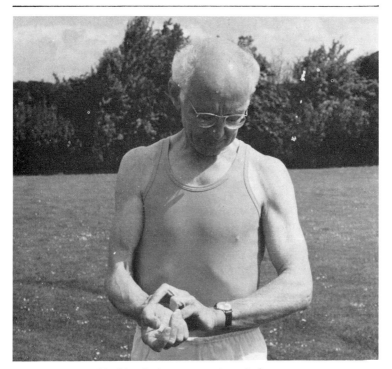

Checking the heart rate at the end of a run.

the guidelines from Table 5.5, you should strive gradually to increase your session to one hour (with the rate of progression based upon HR and perceived exertion). We argue that, to achieve adequate levels of the components of physical fitness most important to health and personal well-being, you should try to devote three hours each week to exercise. And, although this may provide considerable hardship for some (usually the busiest need it most), consider the benefits!

Let us evaluate alternatives to the three days per week training regimen. Based upon experience with people missing one day a week in our adult fitness programme, we believe that two days a week is of considerable benefit — certainly for the sedentary individual of less than average aerobic power[2]. However, three days per week is better. Unfortunately, one day per week may be counterproductive. It is probably better for the over thirty-five sedentary adult to do *no* exercise than to go off to the squash court once a week.

---

[2] It may also be said that one to two hours per week of the exercise described would be of considerable benefit — three hours per week is an idealized goal.

Table 5.5 Guidelines found successful in the prescription of exericse for healthy adults

Measure of Exercise Intensity Following Exercise		Exercise Prescription
HR	**RPE**	
<70% of HR max	11 or less	"Increase" intensity, duration, or both.
70–85% of HR max	12–14	"OK"; increase intensity once a month, usually in five second increments for each ¼ mile; increase duration once a week, usually one extra ¼ mile lap for each increase.
85–90% of HR max	15	"Beware." Check heart rate. Make sure that you are running at the assigned velocity.
>90% of HR max	>15	"Decrease" the intensity, duration or both. Make sure that you are running at the new (slower) rate.

Many individuals may wish to exercise more than three times per week. We are in favour of this, with a few caveats. It is true that the more you run, the more calories you will use and the greater will be the benefits in weight loss and toning of the body. However, in terms of aerobic power, there is clearly a limit on how much you can improve. Beyond a certain point, perhaps six months to a year of the programme, there are going to be very few benefits in terms of extra aerobic power.

There are possible negative consequences from too much running. We have already discussed the danger of 'overuse' injuries. Unfortunately, most daily runners (running five continuous miles and more) 'break down' with orthopaedic problems sooner or later. In contrast, for most individuals who exercise only one hour per day, three days per week, while making an attempt to counteract the possibility of injury with the preventive measures discussed earlier, the risk is minimal.

Michael Sachs, of Florida State University, has recently completed some interesting research in which he identified a 'positive addiction' associated with many distance runners. He notes that some runners develop such a need for running that if they stop for even a day or two, they experience withdrawal symptoms not unlike those of someone who goes 'cold turkey' off cigarettes.

We are ambivalent on the issue of too much running. Our experience has taught us that the overwhelming majority of people who participate in regular systematic exercise grow to love it. Try the three-day-per-week plan described in this chapter. It is all the exercise you really need. If you are a beginner, you will not have to worry about this issue for some time anyway then, after a few months to a year, if you are looking for a new hobby — with lots of expenditure of time — daily running might be for you.

Progression

The first day's exercise programme is an informed hunch. From then on your individualized programme is far more scientific. Table 5.5 outlines a plan for you to follow. Its basic idea is to proceed slowly with your exercise programme. Gradually, increase the number of repetitions for each of your flexibility and toning exercises. A guideline may be to add one extra repetition of each exercise every two training days. For the stimulus period, you generally want to add one or two minutes of running every week.

The progression depends upon your personal response. If you find yourself within the intensity limits already prescribed, progression is a matter of good judgment. For those who begin at intensities H and I, it is good sense to add only a half-minute each week. For those at intensities D to G, a one-minute increment may be more appropriate. A sample progression using the methods described here is found in Table 5.6. Progress slowly and let each day tell you how you are doing.

We would also strongly recommend that you keep a personal record of your exercise programme. Be sure to record your type of exercise, duration, speed, heart rate and perceived exertion each day. Little personal comments may also be useful. Such a record provides a marvellous motivational device as you continue to improve.

Cool-down

An often overlooked point is that following a run (or any other aerobic activity), it is important to close with a five to ten-minute cool-down period. Always finish off your exercise with several minutes of walking. Following the walk, you may incorporate a few of the mild stretching exercises shown in Figure 5.3 (see also chapter 7). And do not forget to do your static stretches from Figure 5.4.

There have been cases where people standing in one place, following a stimulus period, have collapsed. Standing under a shower immediately after a run would be a perfect example. You will remember from

Table 5.6 A daily record sheet for the prescription of exercise with sample progression of intensity and duration, each based on the previous days HR and RPE.

Date	Lap Time (sec) For ¼ mi track	Training Intervals	Post-exercise HR	Post-exercise RPE
Monday, Week 1, Month 1	75[1]	2–1, 2–1, 2–1*	152	13
Wednesday, Week 1, Month 1	75	2–1, 2–1, 2–1	148	12
Friday, Week 1, Month 1	75	2–1, 3–1, 2–1	148	12
Friday, Week 4, Month 1	70	2–1, 3–1, 2–1, 2–1	156	13
Friday, Week 8, Month 2	65	3–1, 4–1, 3–1, 3–1	152	14
Friday, Week 12, Month 3	60	4–1, 4–1, 4–1, 4–1	148	13

[1] These initial values are based on age, sex, weight, recent history of exercise (Table 5.2)

chapter 3 that the leg muscles serve as a second pump for the blood by contracting against the large veins, thus sending the blood back to the heart. If there has recently been a lot of blood pumped by the heart, the blood needs help in going back 'up the hill' from the feet and lower legs. This blood will pool in the veins of the legs if the leg muscles are not being used. If blood pools in the legs, there will be a shortage of blood returning to the heart, which will in turn mean too little blood will be available for the rest of the system. This can mean lack of blood and consequently lack of oxygen for the brain, resulting in a black-out or in lack of oxygen for the heart, which could cause a heart attack. Do the wise thing. Be sure to cool down gradually following exercise.

ALTERNATE FORMS OF AEROBIC EXERCISE

This chapter has been devoted to the run/walk as the best and most efficient means of obtaining the most benefits from your training. We wish to note, however, that it is perfectly appropriate and even wise to insert alternate forms of exercise into your weekly programme. Perhaps, once a week you might enjoy a bicycle ride in the country. You may have access to a swimming pool which makes this excellent aerobic activity available for your programme. Maybe you enjoy continuous dancing to music. Or you might live in a snow region where cross-country skiing is available. Alternatively, you may possess one of the many sports skills which make aerobic activity more enjoyable for some — for example, handball, basketball, squash, soccer, tennis, badminton.

The rules are still the same. Start slow, and do not overdo it. Evaluate yourself by heart rate and perceived exertion. You may be able to work longer periods at lower levels of heart rate and perceived exertion, for example, during cycling, dancing, etc. Do not forget about the importance of warm-up and cool-down. In addition, be sure to consult an expert about safety factors in new activities.

SPECIAL CONSIDERATIONS FOR THE FEMALE

We can summarize this section by saying that there are few special considerations for females. Certainly with regard to exercise frequency, intensity, duration and progression, the rules are all the same for both sexes. While it is true that most research studies tend to show that the average female has approximately thirty per cent less aerobic power than her male counterpart[3], much of this difference must be blamed on western culture where it is often considered 'unladylike' to sweat.

We published a study a few years ago in which it was shown that college women could make up over 2/3 of the difference, i.e. get within ten per cent of a male control group after just eight weeks of exercise. In a recently published study we described young women fully fifty per cent higher in aerobic power than the average American male. There is no question that women obtain the same benefits from aerobic training as do men.

For the beginning of an exercise programme perhaps a few issues which only concern females should be raised. Some women runners require specially constructed exercise bras. With the proliferation of female exercisers most manufacturers now produce those bras which provide for greater support and comfort during running.

Gynaecological problems do exist in a few women. There is evidence to show that exercise during the menstrual period can result in abnormal

---

[3]Certain differences may make it impossible for the average woman to have the same aerobic power as the average man. The most important of these is that women necessarily carry around more dead weight (in form of fat) than do men. Women also have less haemoglobin, blood volume and heart volume than do men.

cramping and pain in some women[4]. On the other hand, many women have won Olympic gold medals during their menstrual period! The lesson to be drawn is that exercise during menstruation is a matter for the individual. You should know your body better than anyone. For most women, vigorous aerobic exercise is perfectly appropriate at all times of the month.

The overwhelming majority of doctors now recommend and endorse the exercise we have described during pregnancy. An efficient circulatory system and strong abdominal muscles are exactly what is needed to bring a healthy baby to term with as little discomfort for the mother as possible. Only during the last few months need your exercise programme be lessened. But be sure to consult your doctor.

In summary, it is safe to say that sex differences relative to the principles set forth in this chapter are minimal. The few differences which do apply to women in no way negate their need for, nor the joy obtained from, exercise.

SOME FINAL PRECAUTIONS

In closing, it should be noted that exercise of the type recommended here is extremely safe. We have never witnessed a heart attack (although we have seen some of the following danger signs). However, it should be pointed out that exercise can provoke certain manifestations of already present circulatory problems. If you currently have one or more of the symptoms which make exercise more dangerous (and which only your doctor can diagnose), you should be aware of certain danger signs.

Your exercise programme is too strenuous if you have not recovered to a heart rate of less than 100 within fifteen minutes following the cool-down. Within one hour you should recover to your normal sitting daytime heart rate — it is a good idea to check this before the programme begins.

Several symptoms call for a visit to your doctor. You should never have to experience a prolonged period in which you cannot seem to get your breath. Dizziness, unusual chest pains and nausea are certain signs that you have overdone it. Check with your doctor!

---

[4] We have refrained from a discussion of the condition known as secondary amenorrhea experienced by certain female athletes who train vigorously and lower their body fat below fifteen per cent, for example, running fifty miles per week. According to some studies, as many as fifteen to twenty per cent of such athletes experience abnormal menstrual periods or no menstrual periods at all. Thus, ovulation does not occur. Reports show that with cessation of heavy training, most of these athletes return to normal menstrual flow. It must be emphasized that such abnormalities usually occur in athletes. Most reports say that normal aerobic exercise improves menstrual regularity.

In contrast, certain after effects are quite normal. You will probably experience some muscle soreness. There are several possible causes. When you have not exercised for a long time, you can easily tear some tiny tissues which wrap the muscle cells into bundles. These tears need time to heal. Also, your blood vessels in the affected muscles may not be capable of getting rid of the waste products of exercise. These waste products, such as lactic acid, may be present for many hours after the actual exercise. As you improve, your circulatory system is better able to handle such materials. Finally, there is the possibility of mild muscle spasm which in turn leads to localized edema (increased fluids) in the muscle — more cause for pain. All of these are normal, but temporary, and are to be expected when you have not used your muscle for some time.

We have already suggested methods, such as gradual warm-up, static stretching before and after exercise, and exercise moderation, which should reduce the degree of soreness. With proper exercise habits such as these, the soreness should be gone within two weeks.

In closing, remember that, for most of us, sedentary life is the more dangerous alternative. Give exercise a try.

SUMMARY

In this chapter we have concluded that the best form of exercise for most people is running. We emphasized that no one over the age of thirty-five should start an exercise programme without first consulting his or her doctor. Also, before undertaking a programme, it is important to purchase a good pair of running shoes.

We have attempted to make a case that exercise should be carried out three days per week, beginning with about thirty minutes per day and working up to one hour per training day. The daily exercise session should begin with a warm-up period, during which you gradually accustom the body to the stimulus phase of the session. During the warm-up period, flexibility and muscle tone may be developed. Tables 5.2 and 5.3 provide a guideline for your initial day's running session. Based upon your past exercise habits, age, sex, weight, and smoking habits, we have tried to give you a set of interval runs at which to begin your programme. It is then up to you to monitor the progression of your programme, based upon HR and perceived exertion. You should progress gradually in your programme, adding time run and speed of run in accord with Table 5.5. Always conclude each day's session with a cool-down period.

CHAPTER 6

STRENGTH

Strength is a very important aspect of fitness. It contributes to power, muscular endurance and sports performance, and consequently is imperative to the athlete. In addition, however, daily tasks such as stair climbing, running for a bus, shovelling snow, gardening etc., require certain levels of strength, and so it is important for us all.

Strength is the pulling force or tension exerted by a muscle during contraction. It is therefore the ability of the body to apply force. Basically there are four types of muscular contraction: isotonic, isometric (or static); concentric; and isokinetic. The differences between them are shown in Table 6.1.

There are three types of muscle tissue: smooth; cardiac; and skeletal. They all have a different structure and function. Smooth muscle tissue contains long, spindle-shaped fibres, situated in various internal organs.

Table 6.1

Type of Contraction	Definition
Isotonic	The muscle shortens with varying tension while lifting a constant load.
Isometric (or static)	Tension develops but there is no change in the length of the muscle.
Eccentric	The muscle lengthens while contracting, developing tension.
Isokinetic	The tension developed by the muscle while shortening is maximal over the full range of movement.

Cardiac muscle is found exclusively in the heart, containing interwoven fibres, while skeletal muscle tissue consists essentially of long, cyclindrical fibres, found throughout the body. It is the latter fibre that contributes to the main force for the movement of the skeletal system. Each of these types of muscle tissue responds to strength training, as follows:

1 *The overload principle*, which states that for a further improvement in strength gains to occur, the muscle must be loaded beyond its previous capacity. For example, if you are weight training you simply lift heavier weights.

2 *Progression* is of great importance. You progressively apply the overload principle, so that your muscle ligaments, tendons, joints, etc., have time to respond in a safe and normal manner. If you are weak you cannot become a stronger person in the space of a few weeks.

3 *Specificity of training* must be considered. If you lift the heaviest possible weights for a few repetitions, you will improve your strength in the muscle groups exercised, whereas if you lift light weights and undertake many repetitions you will improve the *endurance* capacity, of the exercised muscles.

If you are not physically fit (that is having exercised regularly for at least several months) then you should aim to improve your circulorespiratory fitness initially by the progressive exercise programme suggested in chapter 5. When you are fit your body is better able to stand the added stress of applying considerable force to your frame. An individual who is unfit is more likely to suffer injury if suddenly exposing his or her weak body to unaccustomed strain. In essence you need to have adequate circulatory fitness before you undertake any strength training programme.

METHODS OF INCREASING STRENGTH

You can become stronger by using one of the following methods:

1 Strenuous types of athletic performance in a variety of events.

2 Heavy resistance exercise such as weight lifting (isotonic).

3 Resistance exercise against body weight, i.e. sit ups and pull ups.

4 Isometric contractions where a static body position is held against a fixed resistance. You can try this by clenching the hands, holding them parallel to the ground and attempting to pull the elbows or arms apart while still clenching the hands.

5 Isokinetic exercise (see page 80). Using this method, you exercise on an isokinetic machine. The machine enables the muscle to contract at a maximum force at all times.

Research indicates that isokinetic exercise is probably the most effective way to develop strength, followed by isotonic, and isometric

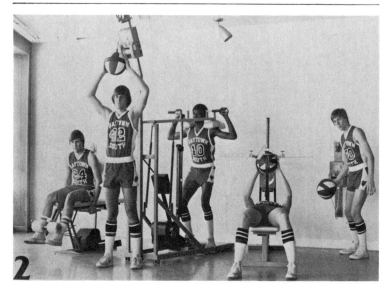

Isokinetic basketball circuit.

programmes. Obviously, strength that is developed by strenuous athletic performance, such as running or throwing events, rarely loads the muscle to extremes and consequently only limited gains in strength can be achieved.

Isometric exercise, although it results in gains in strength, does have certain disadvantages such as increasing pressure in certain regions of your body. This can be particularly dangerous, even fatal, if you suffer from any heart disorder. The authors strongly recommend that if isometric exercise is undertaken maximum contractions should only be held after following a progressive isometric routine for approximately ten weeks. For the individual interested in improving his strength and without access to weights or isokinetic machines, resistance exercises against body weight are probably more desirable and enjoyable. Different schedules for the various strength methods discussed will be explained. It is also possible to increase strength by overloading, for example, by wearing boots or carrying packs etc., while running, but again large strength gains cannot really be achieved by this method. Finally, a combination of strength training methods may be used at the same time (such as isotonics combined with isometrics), but this is not recommended for the man or woman who merely wants to be fit and possess sufficient muscular strength to cope with routine daily demands.

GUIDELINES IN ESTABLISHING A STRENGTH TRAINING PROGRAMME

1 Study the movement pattern of the event or activity and ascertain which major muscle groups are involved.

2 Select suitable exercises to improve the strength of these major muscle groups.

3 Perform the correct number of sets, repetitions, and rest intervals for the type of strength you wish to develop.

4 Undertake the strength programme either one, two or three times per week, depending on your fitness programme and your aim.

5 Ensure that you breathe correctly during the exercise period. The proper technique of breathing is to inhale during upward movements and exhale on the downward movements of each repetition. In other words, breathe in during the initial parts of a movement or contraction, hold it until the latter part of the contraction and then breathe out slowly.

6 Warm up both by *general* and *formal* means before you begin your strength programme. General warm ups involve exercising the large muscle groups of the body, while formal warm up means practising the skill involved in the activity. Several minutes jogging, gradually increasing the pace involving some vigorous arm movements progressively built up, will act as a general warm up, and, if using weights, you may well go through your routine initially using only very light weights. In cold conditions your warm up needs to be longer and progressively more vigorous.

It is also advisable when following a strength training programme to cool-down, possibly by several minutes light running. The jogger who is on a running programme and who runs all the way back to his front door and then slumps in an armchair is asking for trouble. By cooling the body down with light exercise the venous return is implemented (blood returned back to the heart more readily), and consequently the recovery process is hastened. Cooling down is probably more important than warming up after strenuous exercise, although obviously both need to be done.

A comparison of isotonic and isometric strength training methods follows:

Isometric	*Isotonic*
1 Motivation generally low.	Motivation generally high.
2 Little circulo-respiratory training effect.	Low circulo-respiratory training effect but higher than isometric.
3 No special equipment or facilities required.	Expensive equipment. Weights normally required.
4 Generally only fair strength gains (one to two per cent per week).	Higher strength gains than isometrics.

5	Generally a joint needs to be exercised at several different angles.	Strength gains produced in spite of exercising at several points in the range of motion of a joint.
6	Recovery from muscular fatigue poor.	Recovery from muscular fatigue better than from isometrics.
7	No improvement in power occurs.	Good improvement in power occurs.
8	In strong isometric contractions oxygen supply to the muscles is occluded.	Good oxygen supply to the muscles, therefore oxygen supply generally adequate.
9	A rise in diastolic blood pressure occurs during isometric contractions.	No rise in diastolic blood pressure.
10	Minimal muscular endurance effect.	Good muscular endurance effect.

It can be concluded that a higher level of strength can be achieved by isotonic methods than through isometric exercises.

Isokinetics

Faster and greater strength gains can be achieved by this form of exercise. A greater number of muscle fibres are involved with this type of strength programme. Besides being quicker and safer than using weights, little or no muscle or joint discomfort is experienced following an isokinetic strength routine. It is also claimed by some lifters that they do not require a warm up with their isokinetic routine. For rehabilitation following injury, and strength training in general, isokinetics has proved to be the best method of all. In many sports where power is a major factor (such as canoeing, rowing, throwing events, certain gymnastic movements and sprinting) isokinetic strength programmes should definitely be used. This is because the isokinetic contraction will improve the quality of certain muscle fibres which are crucial to the power events. These fibres are capable of strong powerful contractions and cause muscles to move faster.

Types of Exercise

For most individuals a well balanced programme is desirable, and exercises should cater for both the upper and lower body.

O'Shea recommends the following selection and order of exercises:

Monday	*Wednesday*	*Friday*
Bench Press	Incline Press	Same as Monday
Power Clean	Parallel Bar Dip	
Full Squat	Upright Row	
Pullover	Incline Dumbbell Curl	
Sit up	Shoulder Shrug	
Toe Raise	Hack squat	
	Back Hyperextension	

Fig. 6.1   Strength exercises

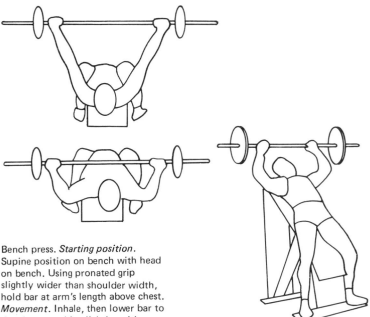

Bench press. *Starting position.* Supine position on bench with head on bench. Using pronated grip slightly wider than shoulder width, hold bar at arm's length above chest. *Movement.* Inhale, then lower bar to the chest touching lightly; with a vigorous arm, shoulder, and chest drive (no bounce or heave permitted), press to the starting position and exhale. When bench pressing maximum or near maximum loads, lower the bar slowly so as to permit complete control of the weight at all times. Throughout the pressing movement, the buttocks must remain in contact with the bench, with the elbows positioned either in at the sides or pointed outwards, practice will determine the most comfortable position. *Major muscles exercised*: (bench press and incline press) 1. Anterior deltoids — P.M. 2. Upper and middle pectoralis major — P.M. 3. Latissimus major — Asst. 4. Triceps — P.M.

Incline press. *Starting position.* Clean bar to chest and then carefully step back to incline bench. *Movement.* Use the same technique as in the bench press, except that at the start of the incline press the bar will be on the chest. The initial press gets you to the extended arms position, which, as in the bench press, is the starting point. Remember that inhalation takes place when you are in the starting position. *Major muscles exercised* (bench press and incline press): 1. Anterior deltoids — P.M. 2. Upper and middle pectoralis major — P.M. 3. Latissimus major — Asst. 4. Triceps — P.M.

81

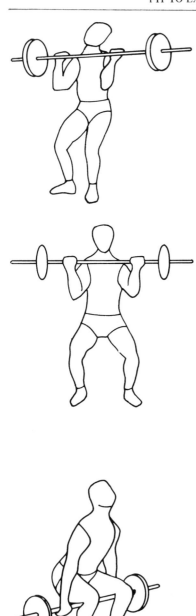

Power clean. *Starting position*. Position the shoulders forward of bar with body in squat position, that is, thighs are approximately parallel to floor, and feet are 8 to 12 inches apart. Hands are shoulder width apart, grip alternating or pronated; arms are straight. Head is up, and back is at a 25 to 30 degree angle, flat, and arched at the base. *Movement*. The initial pull, supplied by the legs and hips, is strong and slow. As the bar passes 4 to 5 inches above the kneecaps, accelerate the pull by extending on the toes and driving the hips upward and forward. Throughout this 'second' pull, raise the elbows high and out to the sides and keep the bar close to the body. At the top of the pull, with the bar approximately chest high, duck quickly under the bar by bending the legs and whipping the elbows under to catch the weight. When power cleaning heavy weights, move the feet slightly out to the sides at the top of the pull.

Once the bar is fixed on the chest, stand erect for completion of the lift. On the initial pull *do not* jerk the bar off the floor by bending the arms and straightening the legs. Always keep the back flat and arched at the base. *Major muscles exercised*: 1. Quadriceps — P.M. 2. Glutaeus maximus, hamstrings — P.M. 3. Erector spinae — Asst. 4. Abdominal and hip flexors — Asst. 5. Deltoids — P.M. 6. Trapezius, upper — Asst. 7. Biceps — Asst. 8. Radial flexors — Asst.

Hack squat. The technique is the same as for a regular squat except that the bar is held behind the legs and the heels are elevated on a block. This exercise may also be performed on a 'Hack machine'. *Major muscles exercised*: 1. Quadriceps — P.M. 2. Glutaeus maximus, hamstrings — P.M. 3. Erector spinae — P.M.

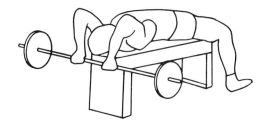

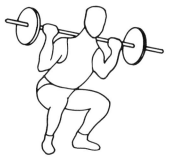

Pullover, with bent arms. *Starting position*. Supine position with head hanging over the end of bench. Pronated grip. *Movement*. Keeping the elbows flexed and close to the head, pull the weight from the floor over to the chest and return to starting position. *Major muscles exercised*: 1. Posterior deltoids — P.M. 2. Lower pectoralis major — P.M. 3. Latissimus dorsi — Asst. 4. Serratus anterior — Asst.

Squat (deep-knee bend). *Starting position*. Bar resting across shoulders, head up, back flat, small of back arched, feet spaced 12 to 14 inches apart. *Movement*. Inhale deeply and squat slowly to a position at which the tops of the thighs are parallel to the floor. From this squat position drive upward, remembering to *keep the lower back arched* and fixed throughout the movement. Rounding the back places great stress on the vertebrae, which can result in serious injury. The squat is an excellent exercise for strengthening the ligaments of the knees, but avoid placing unnecessary strain on them by 'bouncing' out of a low squat position. As an added safety measure, you may use a bench allowing you to squat parallel. If you find difficulty in maintaining balance, you should try the exercise with a block placed under your heels. *Major muscles exercised*: 1. Quadriceps — P.M. 2. Gluteaus maximus, hamstrings — P.M. 3. Erector spinae — P.M.

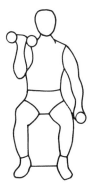

Dumbbell curl (not inclined). Dumbbell curls may be performed simultaneously or alternately from a standing, seated, or inclined position; the last is the most effective position for biceps development. Keep the palms of the hands forward during the execution of the exercise. *Major muscles exercised* (two-hands curl and dumbbell curl): 1. Biceps — P.M. 2. Radial flexors — Asst. 3. Brachioradialis — P.M.

83

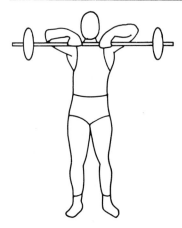

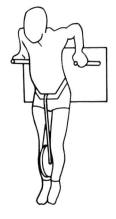

Upright row. *Starting position.* Pronated grip, hands almost touching, arms extended. *Movement.* Lift the bar up to the chin, keeping the elbows high and keeping the bar near the body. On the downward movement, do not let the bar drop without resistance. *Major muscles exercised*: 1. Trapezius — P.M. 2. Middle deltoids — P.M. 3. Biceps — Asst. 4. Brachioradialis — Asst. 5. Brachialis — Asst.

Parallel bar dip. *Starting position.* Arms supporting the body in suspended position between the parallel bars. *Movement.* Dip downward as far as possible and return to the starting position. Avoid unnecessary body swing. You can add resistance by using a belt with a short chain weight. *Major muscles exercised*: 1. Deltoids — P.M. 2. Triceps — P.M. 3. Pectoralis major, sternal — P.M. 4. Latissimus dorsi — Asst. (stabilizer) 5. Radial flexors — Asst.

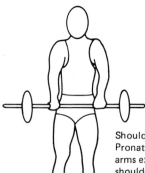

Shoulder shrug. *Starting position.* Pronated or alternating grip, with arms extended. *Movement.* Shrug the shoulders vigorously up and back, breathing deeply. *Major muscles exercised*: 1. Trapezius (upper) — P.M. 2. Latissimus dorsi — Asst.

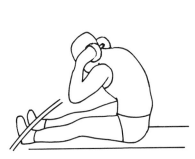

Sit-up. *Starting position*. Hook-lying position, legs bent at knees, hands behind head supporting a weight. Whether in long-lying or hook-lying position, activity of the hip flexors is increased when the feet are held down, and activity of the abdominals is increased when they are not held down. *Movement*. Sit up, touching elbows to knees. Curl back down to starting position. A trunk twist may be added by touching one elbow to the opposite knee. Adding resistance to such a twist brings all of the trunk rotators into action. *Major muscles exercised*: 1. Abdominals — P.M. 2. Obliques, external and internal — P.M. 3. Sternocleidomastoid — Asst.

Back hyperextension. *Starting position*. Prone position, upper trunk unsupported over edge of table, partner sitting on legs. Hands are locked together behind head or holding a weight behind head. *Movement*. Bend downward from the waist until head points toward floor. Return to the starting position arching the back as high as possible. Try holding this arched position for a 2- or 3-second count. *Major muscles exercised*: 1. Erector spinae — P.M. 2. Glutaeus maximus, hamstrings — P.M. 3. Abdominals — Asst.

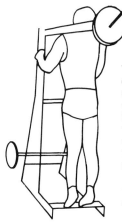

Toe raise. *Starting position*. This exercise may be performed using either a 'calf machine' or a bar across the shoulders. Feet should be 6 to 8 inches apart. *Movement*. Rise up on the toes, concentrating on full extension. Hold this position for a 2-second count. The calves respond slowly to exercise and therefore require much hard work. Repetitions of 15 to 20 are recommended. *Major muscles exercised*: 1. Gastrocnemius — P.M. 2. Soleus — P.M.

85

Weight to be lifted

Following several weeks on a strength programme (without weights), i.e. push ups and sit ups, and when the muscles have become conditioned, then weights may be used as part of the strength training programme. You should not begin with heavy weights. The initial weight used should be the weight an individual can lift for twelve repetitions. Each week heavier weights can be lifted but the increase should be progressive, and the desired objective of lifting heavy weights should not on any account be rushed.

Repetition and sets

A repetition is the number of consecutive times a particular movement may be performed, whereas a set is the number of groups of repetitions of a particular movement pattern.

Research studies generally indicate that for the development of strength one to three repetitions for three to four sets with maximum load is best; for muscular endurance ten to twelve repetitions for three to four sets with maximum load is the most effective; while for the development of strength and endurance simultaneously five to six repetitions of three to four sets with maximum or near maximum load is desirable.

Safety factors when using weights

In lifting weights from the ground, remember the following points:
1 The collars on the weight to be lifted need to be checked for tightness and, if lifting heavy weights, spotters should be used.
2 Feet should be parallel, shoulder width apart and toes close to the bar.
3 The head needs to be held erect.
4 The back needs to be kept flat.
5 The hips should be lowered by flexing the knees.
6 The correct breathing technique needs to be adopted (see page 79).

STRENGTH EXERCISES FOR WOMEN WITHOUT WEIGHTS

The following strength exercises for women are recommended. The number of repetitions and sets will depend upon your physical condition, but initial recommended numbers are given for specific exercises.

Arm and shoulder muscle strengtheners

Initially bend your arms slowly, lower your body until your chest just touches the ground and then return to original starting position. This exercise may be done initially with both knees on the ground, but as your arm and shoulder muscles improve both knees may be placed off the floor when doing the exercise. Also, if you narrow the distance between your knees and hands with knees on the floor the exercise is easier to do, and it is suggested you start the exercise with a narrow base. Do this exercise without pausing. Start with four repetitions and gradually build up.

Abdominal strengthener (1)
From a back lying position with the back of the head resting on the floor, raise your head and chest until, with straight arms, your finger tips touch the top of your knee caps, and then return to the starting position. If you cannot touch your knee caps then reach forward as far as is comfortable with your hands. The back of your knees should be four inches off the ground. Do this exercise without pausing. Start with six repetitions and as your strength improves gradually increase the numbers of repetitions.

Abdominal strengthener (2)
From a back lying position with arms lying by your side and palms flat on the ground, keeping your legs straight, raise both legs together four to six inches from the ground, hold momentarily and lower. When your abdominal muscles are strong enough you may hold the position for

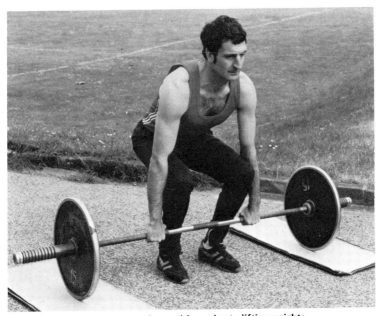

The correct starting position prior to lifting weights.

87

four to six seconds, before lowering your legs. Start with four repetitions and gradually build up.

Leg strengtheners (general musculature in both legs)
From a standing position facing an eighteen inch bench, step on and off the bench straightening both legs as you stand on top of the bench. Repeat this exercise until your legs feel reasonably tired.

Develop muscles on outside of leg
From a side lying position raise the uppermost leg upwards twenty times towards the ceiling. Lie on the opposite side and repeat. Do this exercise slowly without pausing.

Upper back strengthener
Lying face down, hands clasped behind the neck, slowly raise the chest and head off the ground to give an arched position of the upper back. Hold this position for two to four seconds and then gradually lower chest to the floor. Repeat until the point of moderate discomfort.

Lower back strengthener
From a face down lying position raise the legs (keeping straight) and chest from the floor to give an arched position with the upper and lower back. Extend to the position of moderate discomfort. Hold momentarily and then lower your body to the floor. Gradually build up the number of repetitions commencing with four.

PHYSIOLOGICAL CHANGES RESULTING FROM A STRENGTH TRAINING PROGRAMME

Many physiological changes occur following a suitable strength training programme, including:
1 An increase in the size of muscle fibres.
2 Inactive fibres are reactivated.
3 An increase in the protein and fluid content.
4 Better capillarization.
5 Less fat contained within the muscle tissue.
6 Increased connective tissue.

It is also believed that glycogen, haemoglobin and phosphocreatine increase following a strength programme.

Besides possessing optimal strength for everyday life, adequate abdominal and trunk muscle strength helps prevent 'backaches', responsible for millions of days absence from work each week. The vast majority of back and neck aches are avoidable. Backache, sometimes referred to as a 'hypokinetic disease', often results from weak muscles which are unable to support the spine in correct alignment: weak abdominal muscles and erector spinal muscles are very often the culprit. When the abdominal muscles are weak, the pelvis is apt to tilt forward, causing an increased anterior curve in the lower back.

Finally one cannot always assume that adequate strength will be developed just by following one's occupation. The authors recently tested a two hour seventeen minute marathon runner who had been running eighty miles per week for several months and his leg strength and power, despite the running, *was only comparable to the average man.* Needless to say, strength is an important component of fitness.

CHAPTER 7

FLEXIBILITY

Flexibility refers to the range of movement in joints, such as in the knee
or spine. Most athletic pursuits require a certain level of flexibility and
this, of course, varies with the physiological demands of the activity.
Sprinters, for example, require good flexibility in the ankle and hip joints
whereas gymnasts and swimmers generally require a high degree of
flexibility in the spine and shoulder region respectively.

As with the potential for endurance and speed some individuals have
innately a higher degree of flexibility than others, but the range of flexibility in both active and less active people can be improved significantly
by the correct programme. Sedentary individuals usually possess a
restricted range of flexibility in many of their joints, often associated
with poorly conditioned muscles which, in the case of the spine, may
contribute to low back pain. It should be appreciated that flexibility
varies from one part of the body to another and can be limited by bone
structure or by the soft tissues. When it is limited by soft tissues,
improvements can readily be achieved by a suitable flexibility programme. Although extremes of flexibility may be desirable for the
dancer or diver they are not required for the normal individual. A
reasonable level of flexibility will help a person to move more efficiently
and to maintain a relaxed body alignment. A certain level of strength
should also accompany an increased level of flexibility. By a suitable
strength training programme, flexibility of various joints can be
enhanced. Good joint mobility helps to reduce the aches and pains that
are accentuated with increasing age. Stiff joints are also subject to more
strain during locomotion than flexible joints. It is generally believed
that specific stretching exercises are particularly beneficial for the treat-
ment of low back pain.

Adequate flexibility for the demands of a particular activity can help
to increase an individual's physical work capacity, give increased resistance to muscle injury and soreness, and therefore contribute directly to

sound health. There is no doubt that millions of hours from work are lost by men and women who have inflexible muscles and joints and associated problems. Although both slow and fast stretching in various body joints are effective in improving flexibility and differ only marginally in gains, the authors recommend slow stretching because: 1) energy cost is lower; 2) fast stretching is more likely to result in muscle soreness; and 3) there is less chance of overextending the various tissues involved. The various general stretching exercises recommended by the authors are illustrated on pages 93 to 96.

Guidelines before commencing flexibility exercises

If you are out of condition and have not exercised regularly for several weeks or longer then you will need to reach a reasonable level of fitness before you begin your flexibility programme. Please read carefully the exercise guidelines in chapter 5 before you start seriously to stress your joints and tissues. Whether your muscles are in a trained or non-trained state, it is advisable to jog slowly for several minutes (length of time dependent upon the weather conditions, longer if cold), until your cardiorespiratory system (heart and lungs) has had time to adjust to the demands of the activity, and the temperature of your body has risen.

If you prepare for action you will be less likely to strain parts of your body, particularly if you are in middle age. It is also important that you breathe as naturally as possible when doing your flexibility exercises. Do not hold your breath as this places your system under unnecessary strain and may in some cases, because of interference of blood supply return to the heart and brain, result in your fainting. If you are going through your flexibility routine outside on a cold day wear a tracksuit or similar garment. Generally, the heavier the workout you are going to undertake the more important your flexibility exercises become. Finally, following your flexibility routine do not wait longer than twenty to thirty seconds before you start your full exercise programme since, if you wait for extended periods of time, your body may become relatively cold again, and you will not be ready for action.

Bear in mind the necessary guidelines before commencing your flexibility programme, and remember that increased flexibility results from stretching the muscular membranes and tendons, and from extending the ligaments and supportive tissues. It is therefore essential that slow, stretching, controlled movements are performed. Bouncing, stretching movements should be eliminated and the flexibility movements performed to the point of reasonable discomfort. As your programme progresses after several weeks, in order to increase further the range of motion, then greater intensity has to be applied. In other words, keep the movement slow but apply greater effort. Although many researchers recommend a daily routine of flexibility exercises, the authors of this book advise you only to do your flexibility routine prior to your exercise programme and following a suitable warm up by running.

If you are exercising four times per week then *four* flexibility routines need to be done. Nevertheless individuals following a strength session with weights should always finish the session with a range of flexibility exercises applied to the major muscles actively used in the strength work out. A warm up flexibility routine is also suggested using light weights prior to any heavy strength training session.

FLEXIBILITY AND SPEED

Anyone interested in running fast requires good ankle, hip, and shoulder flexibility. Increase in flexibility probably results in an increased stride without a reduction in the rate of leg movement, and, at the same time, leads to a decrease in energy expenditure. If the rate of leg movement is kept constant, running speed can be increased by lengthening the stride. Flexibility training is only effective when used as a supplement to sprint training, and not as a replacement for speed work.

For the normal individual who does not require superior levels of fitness, speed is of less importance than endurance fitness but for the top performer in many sports a high level of speed is a necessity. A good example of this is the English National Cross Country Championship where, usually, the first ten positions are taken by athletes who have a very superior endurance capacity but are also capable of running a single mile in approximately four minutes or even less. In other words, 'starts' to comparatively long races (English National Cross Country nine miles) are getting considerably faster and in order to stay with the leaders these (top) athletes require both speed and endurance.

FLEXIBILITY AND CIRCULO-RESPIRATORY ENDURANCE

Recently the authors physiologically assessed an international cross country runner who, because of comparatively short hamstrings, was continually plagued by injury in this region. This runner had not considered the necessity for flexibility exercises to help prevent this problem, and since undertaking static flexibility exercises in his hamstring region no similar injuries have occurred. Where endurance runners have short legs a suitable flexibility programme may add several inches to the stride length and, providing the leg cadence remains the same, better performances will result.

For the majority of men and women following an exercise programme where heart-lung fitness is a necessity, only a few minutes are required before the exercise period to complete a flexibility schedule. Some injuries such as shin soreness and muscle soreness may be relieved by static stretching exercises. Where any muscle soreness is prevalent the affected muscles should be placed in static stretch for a few seconds and, if possible, several repetitions should be undertaken.

FLEXIBILITY AND STRENGTH

People often think that an increase in strength leads to a loss of flexibility. A suitable weight training programme does not cause a person to be 'muscle-bound'.

However, lifting heavy weights will sometimes increase the range of movement in the exercised joints and may cause some restriction in the joints not exercised. Weight-lifters need to analyze which major muscle groups are involved in their workout and ensure that before and after the weight training session the correct flexibility exercises are done.

Some studies have examined both isotonic and isometric strength training methods and found that neither programme had detrimental effects on flexibility. It is also claimed by some individuals that over-flexibility may be disadvantageous to certain performances, for example scrummaging in rugby, but this is largely subjective and not backed by scientific evidence.

FLEXIBILITY PROGRAMME

The following exercises are recommended for males and females of all ages who exercise regularly. When starting your flexibility programme hold the recommended position for three to four seconds. After six to eight weeks hold the recommended position for ten to twelve seconds, and do three sets on each position. Continually change from one body position to another. Rest for thirty seconds after one complete set of all recommended exercises. Remember not to hold your breath when doing the exercises, and extend to the point of reasonable discomfort. Fortunately, once a good range of flexibility has been achieved, gains are only slowly lost.

1 *Lower leg: to stretch the calf muscles*
Stand with toes on a raised object, hold
on for support with arms. Lower heels as far as
possible towards the floor, raise and repeat several
times (heels at no time actually touch the floor).

2 *Hamstring groin and back stretch*

From a steated position with the legs
stretched as far apart as possible and
straight, one of the ankles is held with
both hands and the upper part of the
body is taken towards the held foot.
(Repeat holding opposite side.)

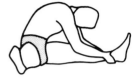

3 *Head rotation*

Stand erect hands on hips, feet twelve to fourteen inches apart. Slowly
rotate the head clockwise in a full circle. Repeat but rotate the head in
the opposite direction.

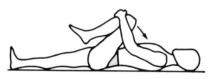

4 *Hip flexor stretch*

From a lying on back position,
slowly pull the knee of one
limb towards the chest,
hands held just below the
knee. Repeat with opposite leg.

5 *Lower back stretch*

Lying on the back, holding each leg below the knee, pull both knees
up slowly towards the top of the chest and hold.

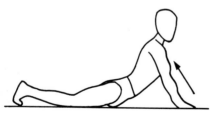

6 *Upper trunk stretch*

Lying on the stomach, push
the upper body back to
extend the arms fully.
Attempt to keep the pelvis on
the floor, and hold head back.

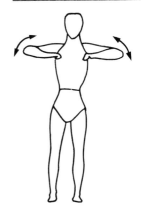

7 *Upper back and shoulder stretch*
Stand with feet twelve to fourteen inches
apart, with elbows bent but parallel to the
ground. Keeping the elbows parallel to the
ground slowly pull them back and hold
in the stretched position. Relax and then
repeat. (Helps to correct round upper back.)

8 *Hamstring stretcher*
Place foot on a chair keeping leg straight.
Take your head towards your knee and
hold. Change to opposite leg and
repeat. (After several weeks use higher
chair.) This exercise can also be done
while sitting on the floor, legs out in
front and together, then forward with
head, placing hands between knees.

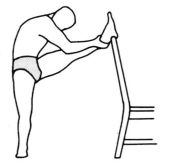

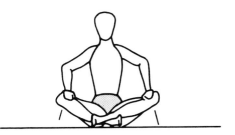

9 *Groin stretch*
Seated and with knees pointed outwards
apply gentle pressure pushing down on the
knees. Release the position and repeat.

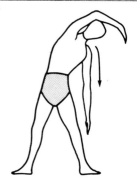

10 *Side stretch*
Standing with feet approximately fourteen inches apart, bend slowly
sideways at the waist and hold in this stretched position. (Repeat
stretching opposite side.) Lift opposite arm to leaning side.

CHAPTER 8

NUTRITION, EXERCISE AND YOUR BODY

Your body is an important source of information, to yourself and to others, about who you are. Social psychologists have drawn a relationship between body image, self-image and self-esteem. In this chapter we will be discussing how exercise and wise eating habits can combine to improve your body and possibly your outlook on life.

For many, the 'social learning' view of the world of Abraham Maslow has great relevance — we are, each of us, trying to become all that we are capable of becoming. This process of self-actualization is clearly dependent upon one's self-esteem. It is almost axiomatic that self-actualization is impossible if we do not like ourselves. And in a society that glorifies the lean body, it is hard to like yourself if you have too much fat.

In some countries, excess fat is common among members of the middle and upper classes. Fat is a sign of affluence, valued as an aspect of personal appearance to be carried with pride. In such cultures, self-actualization is possible for the obese. However, this is not so in most of western society. Our aesthetic values seem to have been handed down from the Greek ideal of the beautiful body. Slimness is a physical characteristic highly valued by almost everyone. This puts a substantial burden on many people. There is a mountain of scientific evidence to show that the obese individual suffers in social situations, is the brunt of constant criticism, fails in job interviews and misses many of the educational opportunities available to his or her slimmer peers. In our society, fat people often have feelings of inferiority, inadequacy, and worthlessness.

Excess fat also has serious health implications. Obese individuals have numerous collateral maladies: for example, hyperglycemia, hypertension, diabetes, cardiovascular and certain chronic pulmonary disorders.

In this chapter, we are concerned with two things: how to get rid of fat if you already have it; and how to avoid it in the first place.

FAT IN PERSPECTIVE

Fat has not always been a disadvantage. It was nature's way of storing energy for a future when food would almost certainly be in short supply. Indeed, fat contains over twice as many calories as an equivalent weight of carbohydrate or protein. Women have about six to twelve per cent greater reserves of fat than men do — probably because of their need to feed a developing foetus in times of want. Probably because of this extra fat, women consistently do better than men in conditions of famine.

How do we make fat and, more importantly, how do we unmake it? The answer lies in a study of evolution. Since the origin of our solar system, the sun has been a provider of the energy needed to do work. One of the truly remarkable evolutionary steps occurred nearly 500 million years ago in the Pre-Cambrian period; green plants developed the ability to trap the energy from sunlight and store it in the molecules of sugar which they produced. Once there was a means of storing the sun's energy, the development of animals was possible. As ecologists are quick to point out, the symbiotic relationship between animals and plants exists to this day. Our body's only way of obtaining energy — energy originally from the sun — is through the ingestion of food in the form of plants, or animals that have eaten plants. In this process of energy transfer (often called metabolism), energy is neither created or destroyed.

ENERGY AND FAT

Energy exists in various forms. It is possible to measure and to inter-convert light, electric, mechanical, chemical and thermal energy. Our body acts as a transducer in converting the chemical energy in food, first to chemical energy in a substance called ATP (the body's energy currency) and then to the mechanical energy of muscular work, heat and/or the chemical energy stored in fat.

The calorie is the most common way of measuring the energy transfer in humans. The calorie is actually a measure of how much heat is given off when food is reduced from a complex form such as fat, carbohydrate, or protein to a simpler form — carbon dioxide and water. An instrument called a bomb calorimeter is available to measure these heat units. Thus, the heat released is the same, whether done in the bomb calorimeter or through metabolism in the body. When you read on the side of a package that one portion contains 100 calories, have confidence in it. The calories in foods listed in Appendix C have all been measured quite precisely!

Almost as soon as we put our food into our mouths we begin to process it for future use. Enzymes in the saliva begin to break down starch into glucose. In the stomach the food is churned into a substance capable of being passed into the blood stream. Once in the blood stream, the food has to be used or stored. If you take in 3,000 calories in a day and only use 2,000, then you will *have* to store the remaining 1,000 calories as fat. *All diets are based on this fact: if you take in fewer calories than you use, you have to lose weight.* The make-up of the diet makes almost no difference. There is a very small advantage in eating a higher concentration of protein as a percentage of the entire diet. But the pitifully few calories saved may cause health problems — and even death — when high protein diets are carried on for several weeks and more. High protein diets are to be discouraged (see page 109).

HUNGER AND FAT CONTROL

It is hunger that tells you when to eat and about hunger some things are still not understood. We know that the control of hunger lies in a tiny, but very important, cluster of cells found in the centre of the brain. This area, called the hypothalamus, is also important for such diverse bodily functions as the sex drive and temperature regulation system. Rat studies have shown that when one portion of the hypothalamus is cut away, the rat will eat incessantly. When another section is removed, the rat refuses to eat anything. Similar results are found when the respective areas are electrically stimulated.

We know that the hypothalamus controls hunger, but we do not know what passes the message along. Whatever the mechanism, it is remarkably accurate. When you eat a few more calories than those needed to maintain weight, you will normally eat fewer calories in the next day or two. You feel just a little less hungry on these days. The effect is to maintain your weight at a fairly constant level. If the hypothalamus was off by just seventy calories per day, i.e., you ate an extra slice of bread per day, you would gain over seven pounds in a year.

Few people have dramatic gains in weight. Weight gain is commonly an extra pound or two per year. All of a sudden you are thirty-five or forty years old and have your personal 'battle of the bulge'.

BODY COMPOSITION

While some people may feel that aerobic power is the most important component of physical fitness, others might conclude that the appearance of their body is just as important. For instance, according to most research, women are much more likely to exercise for reasons of weight control than for other reasons.

As with other human characteristics, the single most important factor in having a beautiful body is to choose your parents correctly. Heredity is crucial. But you can alter the appearance of your body and that is what we will discuss in this chapter. Everyone wants to have the best body he or she can.

Before going further, we will make a brief analysis of those structures which most affect personal appearance. One is the shape of the bones. We refer to the boney superstructure of the body as body type (see Figure 4.3). Like height, body type is inherited — you cannot do a thing about it (except through starvation). If you look far enough into your family tree, you will find someone with a body frame like yours.

Attached to the bones are muscles which have another very important effect upon personal appearance. Muscles have a shape which we can classify as ranging from 'long and thin' to 'short and bulging'. Muscle mass is partially affected by heredity. Also the accumulation of the male sex hormone, the androgens, has a clear effect on overall muscle mass. And, of course, most men have a lot more androgens than most women. The shape of the muscle may also be affected by its position on your bones.

The most important contributor to muscle mass and shape is the amount and type of exercise taken. It is well established that as muscles are used they increase in size and, likewise, when they are not used they decrease in size. The stimulus needed for growth of muscle varies according to your strength (see chapter 6), but even if you do not increase the size of your muscles, systematic exercise guarantees that you will develop a condition called muscle tone. By this we mean a condition in which the muscles are always in a state of partial contraction. Most people would agree that a firm, taut body has a more pleasant appearance than a flabby body with a general lack of muscle tone. Muscle tone is also a source of extra calorie expenditure. So, even as you sleep at night, you will burn a few extra calories as a result of your morning exercise programme.

In addition to valuing a firm body, you may also be interested in its size in absolute dimensions. We have clear ideas, implicitly or explicitly, about what kinds of bodies look good to us. For example, many of us desire narrower waists. As it turns out, a pound of fat does not take up the same space as a pound of muscle. Muscle is more dense and takes up less space than fat.

Following a dance programme at Ithaca College, Kathy Rockefeller found that most of the young women who danced forty minutes per day, three times a week for ten weeks did not decrease in weight. Curiously, however, most reported that their clothes were becoming decidedly more loose. In response to vigorous exercise, the muscles involved were becoming slightly larger and more toned. The difference was approximately an extra pound or two of muscle. The total weight remained the same; that means that these college women were losing fat weight. Since fat takes up a great deal more space than muscle, they had to lose inches.

The next consideration in evaluating body composition (or body appearance) is the skin. Skin colour is, of course, based upon heredity. The skin often takes on an appealing glow following exercise. This is probably a matter of blood flowing to the skin in order to cool the centre of the body. Exercisers seem to have a firm skin. Little is known of the exact mechanisms, but exercise undoubtedly has a positive effect on skin appearance.

Finally, we return to an analysis of fat. The percentage of fat in the body ranges from twelve to twenty-four per cent of body weight in men and eighteen to thirty per cent in women. We describe methods for estimating body fat in Appendix A. We also give a highly subjective method for determining 'ideal weight'. But perhaps the most important way of assessing your fat is to take a good look at yourself, undressed, in a full length mirror.

There is, however, a danger of becoming too complacent, especially if you are young. From about the age of twenty-one, nature and western culture combine against us. At the time when many of us are starting a job which calls for very little activity, an important source of caloric expenditure is lost — we have usually stopped growing. As we earn more money, we can buy more expensive foods which, although often better tasting, are usually high in calories. Nature further compounds the problem by assuring that the number of calories needed to stay alive — the basal metabolism — is reduced with age. In order to keep fat stores constant, we should exercise more or eat less — and we certainly do not eat less. And so many people reach forty or fifty with ten, twenty or more extra pounds of fat.

Throughout various regions of the body, fat stores grow in clusters in spaces between skin and muscles. Unfortunately these fat pads seem capable of nearly limitless expansion, as evidenced by obese persons of four or five hundred pounds. The propensity for expansion seems to be related to the number of fat cells growing in your early years of life. Fat pads are found over most of the surfaces of the body. Most commonly we find them in the area of the abdomen, thigh, buttocks, hips, chest, and back of the upper arm. The specific sites where your fat is stored in greatest abundance is still another aspect of your heredity.

Commonly asked questions about exercise and fat pad accumulation are: How do I get rid of the fat round my waist? How do I get rid of the fat on my thighs? All my fat goes to my hips, how do I get rid of it?

101

The answer is the same for each question.

There is no such thing as the spot reduction of fat. When you lose fat, you are most likely to lose it from the locations where it is in greatest abundance. For example, if forty per cent of your fat is around your stomach, you are, with a ten pound fat weight loss, likely to lose about four pounds of fat from your abdominal region. Specific exercises for a given region are good for toning the muscle in that area; however, they do nothing special for the fat. For the questions raised above, the answer is always the same: jog, swim, cycle, dance, or participate in other aerobic exercises.

We now turn to the most malleable aspect of body composition – body weight. Body weight is simply a function of a caloric balance. In order to gain weight (as you did in your growing years), you have to eat more calories than you use. Weight maintenance depends upon matching calorie intake with calorie expenditure. And, of course, the amount of weight loss depends upon the magnitude of the calorie deficit.

Assuming that you hold exercise habits constant, fat accumulates when your calorie intake exceeds your calorie expenditure. One pound of fat is equivalent to approximately 3,500 calories. Appendix C reveals that you would have to consume an extra thirty-five one-ounce slices of cheese or twenty-three pints of lager before gaining one pound of fat. From this it is clear that fat accumulates slowly.

Unfortunately, the converse is also true. A glance at Table 5.3 on page 66 will reveal that the calorie-per-minute expenditure of a nice steady jog is in the area of about twelve calories each minute. It is easy to see that it will take a lot of jogging to burn off a pound of fat. We should state the principle early and clearly: *Excess weight does not appear overnight and it cannot be expected to vanish overnight.* A corollary principle might be: *For those who do try to get rid of massive amounts of weight in a short time, do not expect to keep it off.*

Some people might interpret the previous paragraph as indicating that exercise has little effect on weight control. This would be wrong – exercise is the sine qua non of weight watching. It helps in several ways. The first has already been alluded to. If you jog sixty minutes a week, according to your size (see Table 5.3 on page 66), you might be expected to use about an extra 750–1000 calories. Assuming that you hold calorie intake constant, this would result in a reduction of about one pound per month, or twelve pounds per year.

This brings us directly to the next point. Not only will you not eat more as a result of a wise exercise programme, but you might eat less. The famous Harvard nutritionist (now President of Tufts University), Jean Mayer, has described a 'critical level' of activity. Working both with animals and humans, he found that a half to one hour's moderate activity will actually result in a depression of appetite. And the timing may be particularly important, i.e., it might help to suppress appetite by participating in exercise as near to your time of eating as possible.

For centuries, farmers have known that they could increase the weight of their cattle and hogs by penning them up. They found that not only do penned up animals eat the same as when left to graze – this alone would result in an increase in weight – but they eat more. Our modern society may be penning us up with trains, cars and lifts.

Another rather recent research finding alludes to the importance of exercise in childhood. There are two ways of gaining fat. One is to increase the number of fat cells, while the other is to increase the fat in existing cells. Two principles have been found. The first is that the number of fat cells is fixed from the age of adolescence. Secondly, individuals with a large number of fat cells in early life seem to have an insatiable hunger and are often obese in adulthood. Obese individuals often have no concept of overeating – they simply eat until they are full. The fat cell theory makes a powerful case for the importance of exercise in the early years of life, with its possible retarding effect on the production of fat cells.

This theory also provides some insight into the rôle of the parent in providing good standards of nutrition for the child. The child should be permitted to eat until he or she is full. The wise parent should provide the child with a wide variety of foods (details to follow) and see to it that the child gets enough exercise.

Leaders of weight control centres are almost unanimous in saying that a successful weight loss programme is nearly impossible without a systematic exercise programme (success being defined in terms of the amount of weight loss and the time that the weight is kept off). The approach of many is to advise a walking programme, and this is very wise in view of the possible orthopaedic problems associated with jogging in the overweight individual. A review of Table 5.3 will reveal that the calorie expenditure in walking a mile is not so much less than in running a mile. For weight (fat) control, distance is the important factor.

The first step in establishing the calorie deficit needed to lose weight is to establish your personal calories to maintain weight (CTM). Following the instructions in Figure 8.1, you will notice that your CTM is based upon your height, weight, age, sex, and of course your activity pattern. Just to be safe – that is, to be sure that you will lose weight – set the food factor at 40. If you eat below the obtained food allowance (CTM), you will certainly lose weight!

An alternative method of determining your CTM depends upon a record of your daily calorie intake over a one-week period (assuming that you are not gaining or losing weight). Simply record everything that you eat. Using Appendix C you can then count your daily calories. The average daily food intake represents your CTM.

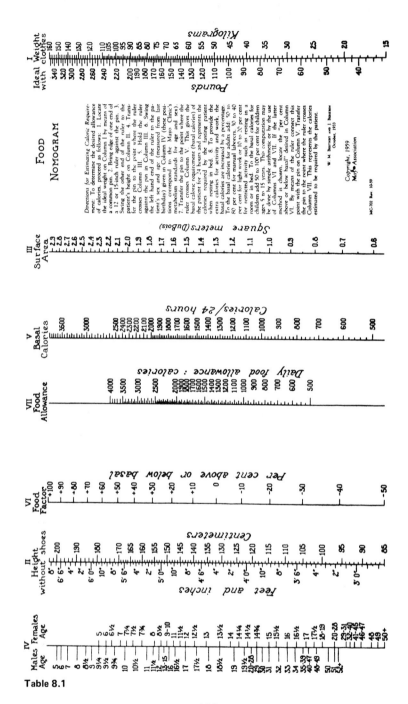

FOOD NOMOGRAM

I — Ideal Weight with clothes — Kilograms / Pounds

Directions for Estimating Caloric Requirement. To determine the desired allowance of calories, proceed as follows: 1. Locate the ideal weight on Column I by means of a common pin. 2. Bring edge of one end of a 12 or 15-inch ruler against the pin. 3. Swing the other end of the ruler to the patient's height on Column II. 4. Transfer the pin to the point where the ruler crosses Column III. 5. Hold the ruler against the pin on Column III. 6. Swing the left hand end of the ruler to the patient's sex and age (measured from last birthday) given in Column IV (these positions correspond to the Mayo Clinic's metabolism standards for age and sex). 7. Transfer the pin to the point where the ruler crosses Column V. This gives the basal caloric requirement (basal calories) of the patient for 24 hours and represents the calories required by the fasting patient when resting in bed. 8. To provide the extra calories for activity and work, the basal calories are increased by a percentage. To the basal calories for adults add 50 to 80 per cent for manual laborers, 30 to 40 per cent for light work or 10 to 20 per cent for restricted activity such as resting in a room or in bed. To the basal calories for children add 50 to 100 per cent for children ages 5 to 15 years. This computation may be done by simple arithmetic or by the use of Columns VI and VII. If the latter method is chosen, locate the "per cent above or below basal" desired in Column VI. By means of the ruler connect this point with the pin on Column V. Transfer the pin to the point where the ruler crosses Column VII. This represents the calories estimated to be required by the patient.

W. M. BOOTHBY AND J. BERKSON
October, 1933

Copyright, 1959
Mayo Association

MC-702 Rev. 10-59

III — Surface Area — Square meters (DuBois)

V — Basal Calories — Calories/24 hours

VII — Food Allowance — Daily food allowance : calories

VI — Food Factor — Per cent above or below basal

II — Height without shoes — Centimeters / Feet and inches

IV — Males Age / Females Age

Table 8.1

104

A final, simple, but less accurate way of determining your CTM can be obtained from Table 8.1. Merely classify yourself by weight and note your CTM. If you measure CTM in more than one way, assume that the lowest value is your true CTM.

We would recommend a slow and steady weight loss programme – about one pound per week. Remember, you did not gain your weight in a few weeks and, if you want to keep it off, you should not try to lose it all in a few weeks.

If you choose to lose one pound a week, that means that you should go on a 500 calorie daily deficit (500 x 7 = 3500 = one pound of fat). Of course, if you are combining exercise with your diet (and we hope that you will), you may also make a few pounds of muscle, thus making an additional improvement in your body by reducing a few inches.

Table 8.1 A quick method for determining your calories to maintain (CTM)

Women		Men	
Weight	CTM*	Weight	CTM*
95–100	1200–1500	120–130	2000–2400
100–105	1275–1575	130–135	2150–2450
105–110	1350–1650	135–140	2250–2550
110–115	1425–1725	140–145	2300–2600
115–120	1500–1800	145–150	2350–2700
120–125	1600–1900	150–155	2400–2750
125–130	1725–2025	155–160	2450–2800
130–135	1850–2150	160–165	2500–1850
135–140	1975–2275	165–170	2550–2900
140–145	2100–2400	170–175	2625–2975
145–150	2200–2500	175–180	2700–3050
150–155	2300–2600	180–185	2775–3125
155–160	2400–2700	185–190	2850–3200
160–165	2500–2800	190–195	2925–3275
165–170	2600–2900	195–200	3000–3350
		200–205	3150–3400
		205–210	3100–3500
		210–215	3150–3550
		215–220	3200–3600

* Depends on your activity level and age. With little activity and increased age the value on the left becomes more appropriate. To ensure weight loss it is always 'safer' to pick the smaller value.

RECOMMENDATIONS FOR A PERSONAL WEIGHT CONTROL PROGRAMME

To begin a substantial weight loss programme, you should first consult your doctor. Only he or she knows the state of your health and how a loss of weight would affect you. It is possible that you will need vitamin or mineral supplementation, for example, it is very common for smaller women to need iron supplementation. Assuming that you do indeed need to lose weight, most doctors will heartily endorse the idea.

The type of diet advocated by Dr Norman Jolliffe in his book *The Prudent Diet* is also recommended. He suggests a diet on an 'every other day' basis. On day 1, you eat 1,000 calories less than your CTM. On day 2, you eat your CTM and so on. Obviously this regimen will result in a 7,000 calorie deficit over two weeks — thus, our one pound per week goal. The Jolliffe diet has several good points. The psychological factor of being able 'to put up with anything for one day', has substantial appeal. Perhaps even more important, the diet assures that weight loss is carried on over a longer period of time than many crash diets. This may have substantial advantages in keeping the weight off!

NUTRITIONAL TIPS

People often ask about what type of foods to eat during a well-planned diet. The answer is very simple: it is important to follow the most up-to-date nutrition research. Every day your diet should contain each of the following food groups: fruits and/or vegetables; milk or milk products; breads and cereal; meats, fishes or legumes.

If each day's diet contains portions of each of these food groups, adequate nutrition is almost guaranteed. One problem can occur with the rather small female who needs to go on a diet of around 700 calories to lose weight. She probably needs to be a little more careful. For her, or anyone who wants to be more careful and scientific about their approach to nutrition, we would recommend the information provided in Table 8.2. This table offers the latest in a series of nutritional guidelines, designed for Americans (but most appropriate for Great Britain), which have evolved since the need arose for feeding soldiers in World War II. Researchers determined what was needed for adequate health and freedom from disease, then they added to that figure. For instance, it was found that 30 mg per day of Vitamin C was all that a thirty-year-old male needs for adequate health and nutrition; they then added 15 to that figure and said that he should have 45 mg of Vitamin C per day.

Vitamin supplementation might be considered when dieting. Of course your doctor should have the last say about this. However, consider that some individuals take 200, 300 and 500 or more per cent of the daily allowances recommended in Table 8.2. In the case of the water soluble vitamins – C and the B complex – the excess is simply passed out in the urine. In the case of the fat soluble vitamins – A, D, E and K – your body can store them. However, too much of these vitamins can be positively harmful. Dr Jean Mayer has reported that certain individuals have even died from going on a vitamin A diet. Clearly, it would take massive amounts of the fat soluble vitamins to kill you, but why take chances with your health? With vitamins, as with most things, too much of a good thing can be harmful.

There are two common fallacies about diets. The first is that starchy foods are fattening. Nothing could be further from the truth. Starchy foods, such as breads, macaroni, etc., contain less than half of the calories found in foods which are high in fats. Appendix C shows that a baked, peeled potato provides only about 90 calories; one slice of white enriched bread provides 70 calories; one four-inch diameter pancake 60 calories; or one cup of spaghetti in tomato sauce with cheese, 190 calories. Starchy foods are *not* inherently fattening (of course any food is fattening taken in excess). It is the oil and butter which we put on the starchy foods that is truly 'fattening'. The dieter must learn to use low calorie oils and only small portions of butter. In the case of spaghetti sauce, the dieter should only use tomato sauce – no oils. It is mainly the fat in the pie crust, not the fruit in the middle, which makes a piece of pie high in calories.

We provide here two lists: of *very good foods* and *very bad foods* for the dieter. Our criteria are nutritional value, i.e content of vitamins, minerals, and essential proteins, and economy of calories. Very bad foods are high in calories and/or relatively lacking in nutrients. You may wish to look through Appendix C to make your own list, based upon your personal tastes and preferences.

Very Bad Foods for a Dieter	*Very Good Foods for a Dieter*
Whole milk dairy products (cheese, whole milk, whipped cream, etc)	Low-fat cottage cheese
	Skim milk
Meat with a lot of fat	Broiled chicken (without the skin)
Fried foods especially chips and crisps	Liver and veal
	Most fish products
Nuts of all kinds	Most vegetables except beans and corn
All pies and cakes, etc	
Butter and margarine	Most fresh fruits
Chocolate	Most soups
Oils	Macaroni and potatoes
Alcoholic drinks	Salads without oils (or low calorie oils)

Table 8.2 Recommended Daily Dietary Allowances,[a] Revised 1974

	Age	Weight		Height		Energy	Protein	Fat-Soluble Vitamins			
								Vita-min A Activity		Vita-min D	Vita-min E Activity[e]
	(years)	(kg)	(lbs)	(cm)	(in)	(kcal)[b]	(g)	(RE)[c]	(IU)	(IU)	(IU)
Infants	0.0–0.5	6	14	60	24	kg x 117	kg x 2.2	420[d]	1,400	400	4
	0.5–1.0	9	20	71	28	kg x 108	kg x 2.0	400	2,000	400	5
Children	1–3	13	28	86	34	1,300	23	400	2,000	400	7
	4–6	20	44	110	44	1,800	30	500	2,500	400	9
	7–10	30	66	135	54	2,400	36	700	3,300	400	10
Males	11–14	44	97	158	63	2,800	44	1,000	5,000	400	12
	15–18	61	134	172	69	3,000	54	1,000	5,000	400	15
	19–22	67	147	172	69	3,000	54	1,000	5,000	400	15
	23–50	70	154	172	69	2,700	56	1,000	5,000		15
	51+	70	154	172	69	2,400	56	1,000	5,000		15
Females	11–14	44	97	155	62	2,400	44	800	4,000	400	12
	15–18	54	119	162	65	2,100	48	800	4,000	400	12
	19–22	58	128	162	65	2,100	46	800	4,000	400	12
	23–50	58	128	162	65	2,000	46	800	4,000		12
	51+	58	128	162	65	1,800	46	800	4,000		12
Pregnant						+300	+30	1,000	5,000	400	15
Lactating						+500	+20	1,200	6,000	400	15

a The allowances are intended to provide for individual variation among most normal persons as they live in the United States under usual environmental stresses. Diets should be based on a varieity of common foods in order to provide other nutrients for which human requirements have been less well defined. See text for more detailed discussion of allowances and of nutrients not tabulated. See Table 1 (p. 52) for weights and heights by individual year of age.

b Kilojules (kJ) = 4.2 x kcal.

c Retinol equivalents.

d Assumed to be all as retinol in milk during the first six months of life. All subsequent intakes are assumed to be half as retinol and half as β-carotene when calculated from international units. As retinol equivalents, three fourths

There is an immense amount of quackery in the diet business. People get rich selling books about every type of diet imaginable, and no type of diet gets more mention than the high protein diet. Such a diet is based on a few grains of truth. First, it is true that we have to take in a certain amount of protein. There are building blocks of cells called amino acids which the body cannot manufacture and which are needed in some quantity every day. Table 8.2 reveals that women need about forty-seven grams of protein each day and men need about fifty-five grams — and that is all! If you are exercising a lot, you may need an extra

Water-Soluble Vitamins   **Minerals**

Ascorbic Acid (mg)	Folacin^f (μg)	Niacin^g (mg)	Riboflavin (mg)	Thiamin (mg)	Vitamin B$_6$ (mg)	Vitamin B$_{12}$ (μg)	Calcium (mg)	Phosphorus (mg)	Iodine (μg)	Iron (mg)	Magnesium (mg)	Zinc (mg)
35	50	5	0.4	0.3	0.3	0.3	360	240	35	10	60	3
35	50	8	0.6	0.5	0.4	0.3	540	400	45	15	70	5
40	100	9	0.8	0.7	0.6	1.0	800	800	60	15	150	10
40	200	12	1.1	0.9	0.9	1.5	800	800	80	10	200	10
40	300	16	1.2	1.2	1.2	2.0	800	800	110	10	250	10
45	400	18	1.5	1.4	1.6	3.0	1,200	1,200	130	18	350	15
45	400	20	1.8	1.5	2.0	3.0	1,200	1,200	150	18	400	15
45	400	20	1.8	1.5	2.0	3.0	800	800	140	10	350	15
45	400	18	1.6	1.4	2.0	3.0	800	800	130	10	350	15
45	400	16	1.5	1.2	2.0	3.0	800	800	110	10	350	15
45	400	16	1.3	1.2	1.6	3.0	1,200	1,200	115	18	300	15
45	400	14	1.4	1.1	2.0	3.0	1,200	1,200	115	18	300	15
45	400	14	1.4	1.1	2.0	3.0	800	800	100	18	300	15
45	400	13	1.2	1.0	2.0	3.0	800	800	100	18	300	15
45	400	12	1.1	1.0	2.0	3.0	800	800	80	10 [h]	300	15
60	800	+2	+0.3	+0.3	2.5	4.0	1,200	1,200	125	18+[h]	450	20
80	600	+4	+0.5	+0.3	2.5	4.0	1,200	1,200	150	18	450	25

are as retinol and one fourth as β-carotene.

e   Total vitamin E activity, estimated to be 80 percent as α-tocopherol and 20 percent other tropherols. See text for variation in allowances.

f   The folacin allowances refer to dietary sourses as determined by *Lactobacillus casei* assay. Pure forms of folacin may be effective in doses less than one fourth of the recommended dietary allowance.

g   Although allowances are expressed as niacin, it is recognised that on the average 1 mg of niacin is derived from each 60 mg of dietary tryptophan.

h   This increased requirement cannot be met by ordinary diets; therefore, the use of supplemental iron is recommended.

ten to twenty grams. But for most people that is easy to accomplish; for example, three ounces of tuna fish contains twenty-four grams. You can use Appendix C to count the number of grams of protein which you ingest in a typical day.

Your body must remove the nitrogen from protein. This takes a very few extra calories. Unfortunately, a diet high in protein for a period of several weeks and more can lead to a condition called ketosis. In this condition ketone bodies are built up in the blood, because of the abnormal amount of fat metabolism deriving from a lack of carbohydrates for energy. These ketone bodies lead to an acidic state, a condition quite similar to one of the symptoms of diabetes. Several Americans have in fact died of high protein diets, and thousands have become ill because of them. Indeed, a lot of the profits from the books on high protein diets go into court costs from liability suits. The daily benefits (above normal diet) of a high protein diet are roughly equivalent to an extra five minutes spent walking, and the risks are too high.

One aspect of nutrition which has gained increasing attention recently is salt intake. We usually take in too much salt. High salt intake has a clear correlation with high blood pressure and therefore with heart disease and strokes. Experts have recommended a salt intake equivalent to 1 to 2 teaspoons per day.

We will close this chapter with a brief discussion of cholesterol, saturated and unsaturated fats. A high percentage of scientists who deal with the etiology of heart disease would say that foods high in cholesterol and saturated fats are detrimental to your health when taken in large quantities. However, these opinions are not universal. There are scholars who are unconvinced of the connection between fats and heart disease.

Perhaps the safest course is to apply moderation. Foods high in cholesterol, like butter, eggs and chocolate, should be eaten only occasionally. Foods high in saturated fats are the animal fat foods such as meat, butter, and lard for frying. Examples of unsaturated fats are fish oils and vegetable oils. They are just as high in calories but they may be better for you, since they have not been implicated in the fatty build-up on the inner walls of blood vessels which can lead to heart attacks and strokes.

SUMMARY

People who think they have all the answers concerning weight and fat control are trying to fool either themselves or you. A basic question remains unanswered as to why some individuals seem to gain weight more easily than others.

This chapter has presented some facts about nutrition on which most competent authorities would agree. The most important of these is that weight is simply a function of calorie intake and calorie expenditure. There are certain aspects concerning your body over which you have no control. You cannot do anything about your height, skeletal frame, or where your fat goes if you gain fat. The task of losing fat, and keeping it off, is difficult if not impossible without exercise of the type described in chapter 5. Even though culture and heredity may seem to be working against us, with knowledge and vigilance we can take off unwanted weight and keep it off.

CHAPTER 9

AGE AND EXERCISE

Even today ageing is a phenomenon which is poorly understood, although it is of tremendous interest to the majority of people all over the world. Most people are interested in such questions as: Can we delay the ageing process? Can exercise play a part in helping to do this?

Strictly speaking, ageing commences with the start of life, and the years of physical maturity are from eighteen to thirty-five. For the purpose of this chapter the authors will concentrate on aspects of ageing and exercise from the age of thirty-five years.

Although many middle-aged and elderly people state they do not feel any different from the way they felt in years gone by, they are, in many instances, made to feel old by the way they are treated. With age the brain loses cells, and with this cell loss there is a gradual diminishing of intellectual abilities in an individual. However, some aspects of intelligence show a steady rise with age, rather than a loss, due to so-called closed systems in the brain (termed 'cell assemblies' by the psychologist Hebb).

In other words, although the brain cells themselves decrease in number with age, because of the more and more complex links which have been discovered to exist between the 'cell assemblies', some of the brain's systems actually continue to develop, although the brain stuff out of which they develop is decreasing in amount. Nevertheless, eventually a point will be reached when intellectual performance begins to diminish. Together with a loss of brain power occurs a loss of vocabulary. As a person ages, trivialities and minor problems may become a cause of irritation or even great concern, whereas the same problems in youth would not have been given a second thought. It is almost as if the brain, functioning with fewer cells, is not able to deal so readily with the problems. As a result of this the individual may begin to worry unduly and in some instances to induce major stress.

With age the skin loses some of its elasticity and becomes more

111

wrinkled, so that by the age of seventy-five the body has shrunk by some two and a half inches in length. At the age of seventy an individual's muscles may be twenty per cent less efficient, twenty per cent less calcium may be present in the bones, heart capacity can be reduced by as much as thirty-three per cent and the efficiency of the lungs may diminish by as much as forty per cent. In addition, with advancing age, eye sight and hearing usually become poorer, as well as balance, and certain heat balance changes occur throughout the system.

In spite of the fact that every human being will age it must be appreciated that the body may have a lot of different clocks. A person may, for example, have a forty-year-old heart, fifty-year-old kidneys, but only a thirty-year-old brain. We are not referring here to transplants, although in the future many new possibilities of rejuvenation of parts of persons will undoubtedly occur, due to medical advances in this field.

It needs to be appreciated that no two individuals have the same physical needs or psychological drives and that chronological age is not the same as physiological age. Athletes such as Jack Foster, the great New Zealand marathon runner, and Roy Fowler, the English middle distance runner, who are both in their mid-forties, are still capable of beating international runners half their age. If veterans such as these are compared with ordinary healthy males twenty or twenty-five years their junior, the chances are that their physiological systems will be in far better condition, and in a sense they could be termed biologically younger, although chronologically older.

In the film world such actors as Kirk Douglas, Charlton Heston and Yul Brynner, who are all in late middle age, are able, because of a suitable life style involving sensible eating combined with exercise, to match feats with some men thirty years their junior. In one of the British National Newspapers recently Charlton Heston, aged fifty-five, was reported to be able to run two miles in fifteen minutes, and does this several times per week. Needless to say such actors as these are still physically attractive and still possess vigour that would shame many a younger man. The point of interest here is that although such individuals are not capable of equalling their previous physical feats of earlier years, their level of fitness has not regressed significantly. With a sensible living pattern and the right amount of physical activity, your level of deterioration throughout middle and old age, could be similarly slowed. It must of course, be acknowledged that some individuals who never take any strenuous exercise may still live to be a good age and still look presentable, but these are genetically lucky, and almost certainly in the minority.

Although we do not know exactly what ageing is, many biologists claim that it involves an 'information loss'. The body appears to 'forget' instructions it once had about self-maintenance. Molecular biological research has shown that the body's 'information' is stored in coded form in the large molecules of DNA, which operate like blueprints. From these, RNA copies are made, like prints from a negative, and these in turn specify the 'machine tools' (enzymes) which carry out all the cell's operations, including the manufacture of more RNA copies. Chemical blueprints, and the copies made from them, are subject to long term damage, in just the same way as man-made products, such as rubber, perish. During the copying process errors are introduced, and these errors might be self propagating, just as faulty machine-tools make faulty products and then more faulty machine tools.

Another theory is that the quality control which the body exercises over the new cells and molecules it makes, may weaken with age. A process such as this could well underlie human ageing. If it does, it might lie in the cells which reproduce continuously throughout life, so that the new cells of an elderly man are different from, and inferior to, those of a baby. It might, on the other hand, lie in the molecular turnover, inside the cells which never divide and cannot be replaced, like those of brain and muscle. One thing that is certain is that, with age, errors quickly accumulate and cells are incorrectly produced. Interestingly, one important sort of cell production leads to cancer, which occurs more frequently during old age.

In extreme old age when mental ability and physical strength are progressively declining, exercise can only play a small part in the act of living, whereas in the early and middle years of old age exercise can be extremely beneficial. Providing strenuous exercise has been regularly maintained into early and middle age, then the human organism will be able to tolerate such a stress with reserve and many physiological advantages will benefit the individual. There should be no age at which a regularly trained, fit individual, accustomed to strenuous exercise, should cease to continue his exercise regime. It may be sensible, however, to cut down on the energy expenditure and the training time spent each day, with each passing decade. Nevertheless, many men and women, even in their eighties still regularly pursue relatively strenuous and enjoyable physical pursuits.

Individuals react differently, even to similar exercise tasks, but where one is under heavy emotional, physical or psychological stress, such as that incurred by the death of a close relative, or by working eighteen hours per day for extended periods of time, then the type and level of exercise needs to be balanced to account for such conditions. Having said this, people in such states may well benefit from programmes of light to moderate exercise prescription.

Accepting that anyone venturing on an exercise programme in middle or old age needs a thorough medical examination, and a medical perhaps twice a year, what then are the benefits of regular exercise?

Firstly, muscular tone is maintained throughout the body, including the heart which will contract more forcefully during both rest and exercise. Secondly, the circulation will be improved, because the aorta and other major blood arteries will have greater elasticity. Good muscular support will help the veins to return the blood effectively to the right side of the heart and varicossities (the pooling of blood) are prevented to a large degree by good muscular tone. A diagphragm possessing good tone aids respiration, or breathing, and through its increased pumping action augments the return of blood to the right side of the heart.

Exercise aids certain psychological states. Many individuals feel they are able to relax more, with consequent relief of anxiety and depression, while jogging, walking, swimming or dancing, etc. Very often a brisk walk with the dog will result in a pleasant, slightly tired feeling which can act as a good base for a sound night's sleep. In fact, it is interesting to observe how well many dog owners look, particularly those who take their dogs for long walks every day. The fact that nervous tension may be alleviated by exercise in all probability aids digestion, as nervous tension all too often is a cause of peptic ulcers. In addition exercise has a favourable effect on bowel function. Suitable exercise can also help to control obesity; if the fat is kept to a minimum in the heart and major blood vessels, then this is very likely to delay, or prevent, coronory death or disability occurring prematurely.

With age, such diseases as emphysema and chronic bronchitis become common and mild exercise within the capability of the individual may well help to lessen such problems. An individual who is accustomed to regular exercise breathes more economically and as a result gaseous exchange across the lungs is achieved more efficiently and consequently such an individual does not need to breathe so regularly. One only has to walk up a flight of stairs with an unconditioned, obese person to hear him gasping for air, to compensate for his inability to process efficiently and absorb the inhaled oxygen. Some individuals are so unfit that one can hear them breathing heavily and gasping for air even while they are using a telephone.

According to Dr Paul Dudley White, the late President Eisenhower's physician, in the presence of any disease, other than in the lungs, suitable exercises can be beneficial. He further states that the majority of patients with heart disease, except for the most severe cases, can benefit by a suitable progressive and regular exercise programme. In fact it is becoming quite common for myocardial (heart) patients, following recovery, to undertake progressive walking, jogging and running programmes, developing, perhaps, over several years. The eventual aim in some cases is to run a full marathon (over twenty-six miles) non-stop.

Although no studies of humans have demonstrated that regular exercise increases the length of life, several studies on rats have demon-

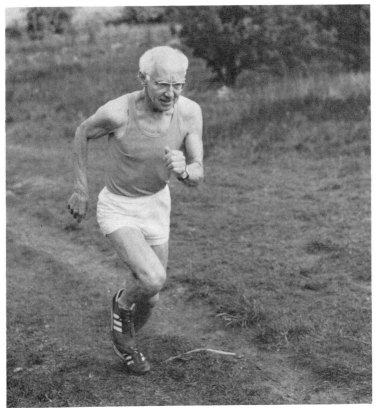

Eric Marsh only started running at the age of fifty-nine and by careful progression he was able two years later to complete a marathon in 3 hours 33 minutes. He is a classic example of what can be achieved.

strated that exercise results in enhanced longevity. It is very likely that regular exercise contributes to the prevention of major cardiovascular diseases and so, indirectly, helps to prolong life. Irrespective of whether life is prolonged, the quality of life will certainly be improved through exercise.

It is of course imperative to start on any exercise programme (partticularly if you are over thirty-five) in a steady, gradual manner, having first received a full medical examination, and the go-ahead to commence your exercise programme. An ideal exercise programme needs to be undertaken for at least thirty minutes, three days per week, and gradually built up to one hour, three days per week. Your emotional and

115

social needs should be balanced with your physical needs, and obviously it is of paramount importance that you *enjoy* the type of exercise you have selected. Rather than just satisfying daily needs, you need to plan your exercise routine for the future, the same way as you would provide for financial security on your retirement.

Many years ago, when I was a member of a boxing club, I remember a distinguished man, in his mid-forties, Squire Dick Burton, training and boxing with younger men, twenty-five years younger than him. In spite of his undoubted skill, his level of specific fitness was exceptional. While recently enjoying a holiday in Shropshire with some friends, I was told of a man in his sixties whom at a local fête, suitably attired with boxing gloves, was taking on all comers and more than holding his own. It was indeed the same man I had boxed with some twenty years before. He had, in fact, kept regularly in training, and is living proof of what can be achieved in later life, for boxing is a physically demanding sport, requiring a very high level of fitness.

How you view yourself (self-image) is very often how you *feel*. If you feel active you can *be* active, and nowhere was this demonstrated more than in Japanese Prisoner of War Camps during the last war, where the men and women who were determined to survive were generally the ones who did. In other words, you must have the will to remain active and young.

Although individuals on similar exercise programmes with similar life styles may age at different levels, a fit middle or old-aged person adds life and vigour to his years, and has a cardiac reserve useful for emergencies. All the available evidence points to the fact that the ravages of old age can be slowed down by a progressive, vigorous programme of physical exercise. Among the sports to be recommended for middle-aged and elderly people are walking, jogging, swimming, ballroom dancing, tennis and cycling.

In conclusion, you must remember that you cannot put back months or years of inactivity in a short period of time, no matter who you are. Any lay-off from vigorous activities must be followed by a period of progressive rebuilding, to regain your former level of fitness. In general, the older you are, the lower your first work load should be, and the longer the period of progressive rebuilding required. In tennis, for example, one may play doubles instead of singles. It is also suggested that during middle and old age you compete or play against individuals of a similar age.

Finally, it is recommended by the authors of this book, that middle-aged and elderly individuals have a full medical examination at least once a year, and preferably twice.

CHAPTER 10

EVALUATION AND TESTING FOR FITNESS

Fitness has several components and therefore it is at present impossible to have one test which encompasses them all. Furthermore, we feel it is necessary to select field tests that are relatively easy to administer, require little or no equipment and relate well to laboratory tests that have been proven scientifically.

It cannot be emphasized too strongly that only individuals who are in good health and are physically conditioned should undertake any form of strenuous exercise testing. There have been cases of individuals undergoing, for example, strength tests (push ups) who have suffered cardiac failure resulting in death. In many instances a reasonable level of fitness is required before a test, for example a running test, can be undertaken safely. Generally, it is advisable to undergo the tests with some reserve and not aim for maximum performance. Maximal capacity tests are more suitable either for the fully trained athlete particularly interested in performance improvement, or for the average individual in a controlled setting, such as a hospital.

REASONS FOR SELF EVALUATION

By undergoing various work capacity tests, your initial work capacity level can be assessed, and later this information can be used as a reference for future comparisons. It is indeed very gratifying to be able to see improvement in your level of fitness, and this can be a source of encouragement for the maintenance of an exercise programme. On the other hand, if an individual does relatively badly on a test, then this can act as a spur to encourage more commitment towards training in the future. The majority of individuals undertaking a fitness programme like to check their progress and testing is one of the best ways to do this.

117

AEROBIC POWER

A foremost American authority on the subject of exercise physiology, Dr Kenneth H. Cooper, suggests that a good test of aerobic power or endurance capacity is the distance that you can cover in twelve minutes by running/walking. Cooper related the maximum oxygen uptakes (VO_2 max in ml/kg. min) of many individuals measured on the tread-mill with physiological measuring equipment, with the greatest distance they could cover in twelve minutes. The relationship between the two was very high (coefficient of correlation 0.89).

It is extremely important that you run and/or walk as far as you can in twelve minutes, but within your present capacity and level of fitness. If you are straining, or feeling distressed, slow down or walk until you get your breath back. At the end of the twelve minutes you should not be distressed or exhausted, but only pleasantly fatigued. In other words, you should exercise within your cardiovascular capacity. In essence, providing you are trained, the higher your maximum oxygen uptake (VO_2 max ml/kg. min) in relation to your body weight the further you should be able to travel in the twelve minute period. Tables 10.1 and 10.2 give the information you require in order to determine your fitness category. As an example, a male of thirty-five years of age covering between 1.57 and 1.69 miles or more in twelve minutes would have an estimated oxygen uptake between 45.0 and 49.4 ml/kg min and be placed in the 'excellent' fitness category.

Besides the twelve minute run test for men and women there is Cooper's 1.5 mile run; the fitness classifications for this can also be taken from Tables 10.1 and 10.2. In each column is the predicted oxygen uptake in ml/kg. min related either to the distance you have covered in twelve minutes, or to your time for running 1.5 miles. If you are neither fully trained, nor in a high state of physical fitness, then we suggest you attempt the 1.5 mile run with the same safeguards we have previously mentioned, rather than the twelve minute test, until your level of condition warrants this. Recently, prior to the start of the rugby league season, we tested the English Rugby League referees on the 1.5 mile run. As they were not fully trained we instructed them to run/walk 1.5 miles, but not at a maximum effort, in other words, relatively fast within their reserve, but not be exhausted at the end of the run.

Humphreys, working with trained college athletes representing the sports of soccer, cross-country running, hockey, and rugby also showed there to be a close relationship between the subjects' maximum oxygen uptake (VO_2 max ml/kg. min) and the distance they could run in sixteen minutes.

Needless to say, we do not recommend individuals to attempt a

118

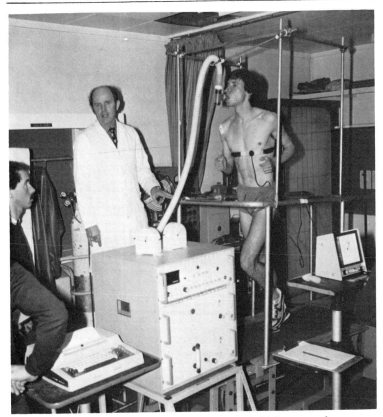

Sebastian Coe being tested by Dr John Humphreys in his human performance laboratory.

maximal performance run for a period of sixteen minutes unless they have achieved a superior level of fitness.

STRENGTH TESTS

Although many tests of strength involve equipment such as dynamometers and tensiometers, these are expensive and in many instances do not measure strength in various muscle groups accurately. Sit-ups and push-ups improve the strength in the muscles of the abdomen, trunk, shoulders, arms and back, and are easy to administer and assess.

Push-ups
Lie face down, with the whole of your body resting on the floor (Figure

119

Table 10.1 Men's aerobics fitness classification (predicted)

Category	Measure	13–19	20–29	30–39	40–49	50–59	60+
I. Very poor	O_2 uptake (ml/kg/min)	<35.0	<33.0	<31.5	<30.2	<26.1	<20.5
	*T. M. time (min:sec,	<14:30	<12:50	<12:00	<11:00	<9:00	<5:30
	12-min. dist. (mi)	<1.30	<1.22	<1.18	<1.14	<1.03	<.87
	1.5-mile time (min:sec)	>15:31	>16:01	>16:31	>17:31	>19:01	>20:01
II. Poor	O_2 uptake (ml/kg/min)	35.0–38.3	33.0–36.4	31.5–35.4	30.2–33.5	26.1–30.9	20.5–26.0
	*T. M. Time (min:sec)	14:30–16:44	12:50–15:29	12:00–14:59	11:00–13:29	9:00–11:29	5:30–8:49
	12-min. dist. (mi)	1.30–1.37	1.22–1.31	1.18–1.30	1.14–1.24	1.03–1.16	.87–1.02
	1.5-mile time (min:sec)	12:11–15:30	14:01–16:00	14:44–16:30	15:36–17:30	17:01–19:00	19:01–20:00
III. Fair	O_2 uptake (ml/kg/min)	38.4–45.1	36.5–42.4	35.5–40.9	33.6–38.9	31.0–35.7	26.1–32.2
	*T. M. time (min:sec)	16:45–21:07	15:30–18:59	15:00–17:59	13:30–16:59	11:30–14:59	8:50–12:29
	12-min. dist. (mi)	1.38–1.56	1.32–1.49	1.31–1.45	1.25–1.39	1.17–1.30	1.03–1.20
	1.5-mile time (min:sec)	10:49–12:10	12:01–14:00	12:31–14:45	13:01–15:35	14:31–17:00	16:16–19:00
IV. Good	O_2 uptake (ml/kg/min)	45.2–50.9	42.5–46.4	41.0–44.9	39.0–43.7	35.8–40.9	32.2–36.4
	*T. M. time (min:sec)	21:08–24:44	19:00–21:59	18:00–20:59	17:00–19:59	15:00–17:59	12:30–15:44
	12-min. dist. (mi)	1.57–1.72	1.50–1.64	1.46–1.56	1.40–1.53	1.31–1.44	1.21–1.32
	1.5-mile time (min:sec)	9:41–10:48	10:46–12:00	11:01–12:30	11:31–13:00	12:31–14:30	14:00–16:15
V. Excellent	O_2 uptake (ml/kg/min)	51.0–55.9	46.5–52.4	45.0–49.4	43.8–48.0	41.0–45.3	36.5–44.2
	*T. M. time (min:sec)	24:45–27:47	22:00–24:59	21:00–23:59	20:00–22:59	18:00–21:14	15:45–20:37
	12-min. dist. (mi)	1.73–1.86	1.65–1.76	1.57–1.69	1.54–1.65	1.45–1.58	1.33–1.55
	1.5-mile time (min:sec)	8:37–9:40	9:45–10:45	10:00–11:00	10:30–11:30	11:00–12:30	11:15–13:59
VI. Superior	O_2 uptake (ml/kg/min)	>56.0	>52.5	>49.5	>48.1	>45.4	>44.3
	*T. M. time (min:sec)	>27:48	>25:00	>24:00	>23:00	>21:15	>20:38
	12-min. dist. (mi)	>1.87	>1.77	>1.70	>1.66	>1.59	>1.56
	1.5-mile time (min:sec)	<8:37	<9:45	<10.00	<10:30	<11:00	<11:15

*Treadmill time using Balke-Ware technique.

Table 10.2 Women's aerobics fitness classification (predicted)

Category	Measure	Age (years)					
		13–19	20–29	30–39	40–49	50–59	60+
I. Very poor	O$_2$ uptake (ml/kg/min)	<25.0	<23.6	<22.8	<21.0	<20.2	<17.5
	*T. M. time (min:sec)	<8:30	<7:46	<7:15	<6:00	<5:38	<4:00
	12-min. dist. (mi)	<1.0	<.96	<.94	<.88	<.84	<.78
	1.5-mile time (min:sec)	>18:31	>19:01	>19:31	>20:01	>20:31	>21:01
II. Poor	O$_2$ uptake (ml/kg/min)	25.0–30.9	23.6–28.9	22.8–26.9	21.0–24.4	20.2–22.7	17.5–20.1
	*T. M. time (min:sec)	8:30–11:29	7:46–10:09	7:15–9:29	6:00–7:59	5:38–6:59	4:00–5:32
	12-min. dist. (mi)	1.00–1.18	.96–1.1	.95–1.05	.88–.98	.84–.93	.78–.86
	1.5-mile time (min:sec)	18:30–16:55	19:00–18:31	19:30–19:01	20:00–19:31	20:30–20:01	21:00–20:31
III. Fair	O$_2$ uptake (ml/kg/min)	31.0–34.9	29.0–32.9	27.0–31.4	24.5–28.9	22.8–26.9	20.2–24.4
	*T. M. time (min:sec)	11:30–13:59	10:10–12:59	9:30–11:59	8:00–10:59	7:00–9:29	5:33–7:59
	12-min. dist. (mi)	1.19–1.29	1.12–1.22	1.06–1.18	.99–1.11	.94–1.05	.87–.98
	1.5-mile time (min:sec)	16:54–14:31	18:30–15:55	19:00–16:31	19:30–17:31	20:00–19:01	20:30–19:31
IV. Good	O$_2$ uptake (ml/kg/min)	35.0–38.9	33.0–36.9	31.5–35.6	29.0–32.8	27.0–31.4	24.5–30.2
	*T. M. time (min:sec)	14:00–17:29	13:00–15:59	12:00–14:59	11:00–12:59	9:30–11:59	8:00–10:59
	12-min. dist. (mi)	1.30–1.43	1.23–1.34	1.19–1.29	1.12–1.24	1.06–1.18	.99–1.09
	1.5-mile time (min:sec)	14:30–12:30	15:54–13:31	16:30–14:31	17:30–15:56	19:00–16:31	19:30–17:31
V. Excellent	O$_2$ uptake (ml/kg/min)	39.0–41.9	37.0–40.9	35.7–40.0	32.9–36.9	31.5–35.7	30.3–31.4
	*T. M. time (min:sec)	17:30–18:59	16:00–17:59	15:00–16:59	13:00–15:59	12:00–14:59	11:00–11:59
	12-min. dist. (mi)	1.44–1.51	1.35–1.45	1.30–1.39	1.25–1.34	1.19–1.30	1.10–1.18
	1.5-mile time (min:sec)	12:29–11:50	13:30–12:30	14:30–13:00	15:55–13:45	16:30–14:30	17:30–16:30
VI. Superior	O$_2$ uptake (ml/kg/min)	>42.0	>41.0	>40.1	>37.0	>35.8	>31.5
	*T. M. time (min:sec)	>19:00	>18:00	>17:00	>16:00	>15:00	>12:00
	12-min. dist. (mi)	>1.52	>1.46	>1.40	>1.35	>1.31	>1.19
	1.5-mile time (min:sec)	<11:50	<12:30	<13:00	<13:45	<14:30	<16:30

*Treadmill time using Balke-Ware technique.

10.1). You then extend your arms into the position shown in Figure 10.2. From this position you bend your arms at the elbow and take the whole of your body in a straight position down until it rests ¼" from, and parallel to the ground. You then extend your body into the position shown in Figure 10.2 again and repeat the movement as many times as possible in two minutes.

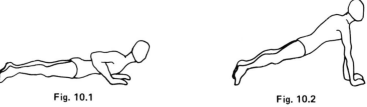

Fig. 10.1   **Fig. 10.2**

Sit-ups

From the initial position of lying on your back with your head and whole body resting on the floor, you bend both knees, so that the backs of your knees are approximately four inches from the ground. You then lift your trunk and head from the ground, keeping your heels on the ground and simultaneously with both hands (finger tips) touch the front of your knee caps and then return to the back lying position. Repeat this movement as many times as possible in one minute. If your abdominal muscles are particularly weak you may place your legs under a chair or bench in order to keep your heels on the ground.

Muscular endurance test standards for push-ups and sit-ups for males and females can be seen in Tables 10.3 and 10.4.

SUBMAXIMAL BENCH STEPPING TEST

The prediction of maximum oxygen uptake can be determined by a submaximal bench stepping test. Usually the person with a lower heart rate will be in better physical condition, and consequently will have a higher maximum oxygen uptake. When taking this test, you step up and down on a bench sixteen and one quarter inches high, for three minutes. The stepping rate per minute is twenty-four for men and twenty-two for women. Step timing is best achieved by using a metronome. Following completion of the test, the participant remains standing while the pulse is counted for a fifteen-second interval, beginning five seconds after completion of the test. To obtain the recovery heart rate to beats per minute, multiply the fifteen-second heart rate by four. The equations for estimating maximum oxygen uptake are as follows:

Men 111.33 − (0.42 x step test pulse rate, beats/min).
Women 65.81 − (0.1847 x step test pulse rate, beats/min).

Table 10.3 Push up muscular endurance test standards(a)

Age	Males					Females[b]			
	Excellent	Good	Average	Fair	Poor	Excellent	Good	Average	Fair	Poor
20–29	55-above	45–54	35–44	20–34	0–19	49-above	34–48	17–33	6–16	0–5
30–39	45-above	35–44	25–34	15–24	0–14	40-above	25–39	12–24	4–11	0–3
40–49	40-above	30–39	20–29	12–19	0–11	35-above	20–34	8–19	3–7	0–2
50–59	35-above	25–34	15–24	8–14	0–7	30-above	15–29	6–14	2–5	0–1
60–69	30-above	20–29	10–19	5–9	0–4	20-above	5–19	3–4	1–2	0

(a) These values are approximations
b Modified push up

Table 10.4 Sit up muscular endurance test standards a,b

Age	Males					Females[b]			
	Excellent	Good	Average	Fair	Poor	Excellent	Good	Average	Fair	Poor
20–29	48-above	43–47	37–42	33–36	0–32	44-above	39–43	33–38	29–32	0–28
30–39	40-above	35–39	29–34	25–28	0–24	36-above	31–35	25–30	21–24	0–20
40–49	35-above	30–34	24–29	20–23	0–19	31-above	26–30	19–25	16–18	0–15
50–59	30-above	25–29	19–24	15–18	0–14	26-above	21–25	15–20	11–14	0–10
60–69	25-above	20–24	14–19	10–13	0–9	21-above	16–20	10–15	6–9	0–5

a These values are approximations
b Test is timed for 60 seconds

Table 10.5 Percentile ranking for recovery heart rate and predicted maximal oxygen consumption for male and female college students.

Percentile Ranking	Recovery H.R. Female	Predicted Max VO$_2$[a] (ml/kg min)	Recovery H.R. Male	Predicted Max VO$_2$ (ml/kg min)
100	128	42.2	120	60.9
95	140	40.0	124	59.3
90	148	38.5	128	57.6
85	152	37.7	136	54.2
80	156	37.0	140	52.5
75	158	36.6	144	50.9
70	160	36.3	148	49.2
65	162	35.9	149	48.8
60	163	35.7	152	47.5
55	164	35.5	154	46.7
50	166	35.1	156	45.8
45	168	34.8	160	44.1
40	170	34.4	162	43.3
35	171	34.2	164	42.5
30	172	34.0	166	41.6
25	176	33.3	168	40.8
20	180	32.6	172	39.1
15	182	32.2	176	37.4
10	184	31.8	178	36.6
5	196	29.6	184	34.1

From F. Katch and W. McArdle 'Nutrition, Weight Control and Exercise' Copyright © 1977 by Houghton Mifflin Company. Reprinted by permission of publisher.
[a] Max VO$_2$ = Maximum oxygen consumption.

A quick way to obtain the proper value is to refer to Table 10.5. However, the standards there are from data collected on college-age men and women, and consequently information collected on middle-aged participants could give slightly lower oxygen uptake values. When you have determined your maximum oxygen uptake, consult Table 10.6 to determine your fitness classification.

Table 10.6

Fitness Classification	Maximum Oxygen Uptake	
	ML/KG MIN	METS*
1	17.5	5.0
	21.0	6.0
	24.5	7.0
	27.0	7.7
2	29.0	8.3
	31.5	9.0
	35.0	10.0
3	37.0	10.6
	39.0	11.1
	41.0	11.7
4	42.5	12.1
	45.0	12.9
	46.5	13.1
5	48.0	13.7
	49.5	13.9
	51.5	14.4
6	53.0	15.1
	55.0	15.7
	56.5	16.1
	58.0	16.6
7	60.0	17.1
	63.5	18.1
	66.0	18.9
	68.0	19.4
8	71.5	20.4
	74.0	21.1
	77.5	22.1

*MET refers to metabolic equivalent above the resting metabolic level. Value at rest is approximately 3.5 millilitres per kilogram of body weight per minute oxygen consumed. The authors of this book recommend that only individuals highly trained and under thirty-five years of age should attempt this test.

HEART AND BREATHING RATES

Although the resting heart-rate may range from fifty to one hundred beats per minute, as a general rule the higher your aerobic power the lower your resting heart rate will be. As your fitness level improves, your resting heart rate will normally be lower. Several international marathon runners have a resting heart rate approaching the low forties. Observation of their resting heart rates indicates when they are reaching a high state of training and are ready to race competitively. The resting breathing rate per minute is normally lower in the trained athlete too and, once again, as you become fitter, so your resting breathing rate is lowered, that is to say you need less air for oxygen exchanged within the lungs and tissues, because your metabolism is more efficient. It is a good idea to record your breathing and heart rate, in bed, ten minutes after you have awakened and note the decrease in these parameters as your level of fitness improves. Both may be recorded for a full minute.

RECOVERY HEART AND BREATHING RATE TESTS

From a standard test of your choice, such as a one-mile run (providing you are fit enough to do this), record your heart rate for fifteen seconds immediately following the run, preferably on the radial artery (wrist), and then multiply by four to convert it to beats per minute. In the recovery period record your heart rate again for fifteen seconds between one minute forty-five seconds and two minutes, and then multiply by four to convert it to beats per minute. Subtract this latter heart rate recovery, from the former, and this is your Cardiac Recovery Index (CRI). As you get fitter, your CRI will be higher because you are returning to the resting state faster. For example, following a one mile run your heart rate after fifteen seconds is forty. Multiply by four to convert to beats per minute.

$$40 \times 4 = 160$$

Heart rate between one minute forty-five seconds and two minutes is thirty. Multiply by four to convert to beats per minute.

$$30 \times 4 = 120$$

To determine your CRI subtract 120 (second recovery index) from 160 (first recovery index).

$$160 - 120 = 40 = CRI$$

If you record your breathing rate, or respiratory frequency (the in and out movement of your chest as can be seen just below the diaphragm), immediately you cease exercise, for the duration of one minute, and denote this as your exercise breathing rate, for example 50 BPM (breaths per minute). Also following exercise when one minute has elapsed record your breathing rate from the end of the first minute to the end of the second minute, then note this figure, for example 30 BPM. Subtract the second figure from the first, i.e. 50–30 and this is your breathing recovery index (BRI). You will note an increase in your BRI as your level of fitness improves, when undertaking the same standard exercise task over a period of time.

APPENDIX A

A METHOD FOR DETERMINING YOUR IDEAL WEIGHT AND TARGET WEIGHT LOSS OR GAIN

Determination of body fat

The most accurate method of determining your body fat would be to immerse yourself in water and directly calculate your density, i.e., the degree to which you sink — fat floats. However, with the use of skinfold calipers you can gain much the same information as if you had been 'dunked' in a tank of water. You may determine your fat weight, lean weight and 'ideal' body weight with the following simple procedure:

1. Using a skinfold caliper, obtain measurement at the following sites:

    Triceps — with the arm resting comfortably by its side, take a vertical fold halfway between the elbow and top of the shoulder — the back of the upper arm.

    Biceps — in the same position, take a vertical fold on the front of the upper arm — just on top of your 'muscle'.

    Subscapular — take a fold on a line parallel with the shoulder blade, just below the lowest tip of the shoulder blade.

    Iliac — take a vertical fold just above the top of your pelvic bone at the side — the area where some have been known to develop a 'spare tyre'.

2. Add these four measurements and find your percent fat based upon the table on page 130*.

3. To determine fat weight, multiply percent fat X total weight.

4. To determine lean weight, subtract fat weight from your total weight.

5. In order to determine your 'ideal' weight, you must establish your 'ideal' percent fat.**

128

6. Based on the considerations cited below, what is your ideal percent fat?

7. Subtract ideal percent fat (6) from 100%, e.g., 100% − 15 = .85.

8. Then:
$$\text{Ideal Weight} = \frac{\text{Lean Body Weight (from 4)}}{\text{Percentage obtained (from 7)}} = \underline{\hspace{3cm}}$$

9. You may go farther and measure your target weight loss or gain as follows: Present Weight − Ideal Weight = _____

   or

   Ideal Weight − Present Weight = Target Weight Gain _____

*Adapted from a table developed by Philip Allsen in *Conditioning and Physical Fitness*, W. C. Brown Co., Dubuque, Iowa. His table was adapted from the work of: Durnin, J. V. G. A. and J. Womersley, *British Journal of Nutrition* Vol. 32, page 95, 1974.

**An individual's 'ideal' weight is clearly based upon aesthetic and cultural considerations. Perhaps the ideal percent fat for a man is between 12 and 15 percent. For a female, the 'ideal' percent fat is 8-10 percent higher or between 20 and 25 percent. Age and the nature of the individual's physical activity clearly alter these considerations. A male marathon runner or wrestler would want to have a percent fat at about five percent or even lower while it is possible to have success in rugby at levels of percent fat higher than the ideal listed above. Similarly, the female runner may need percent fat accumulation of 10-15 percent while her swimming counterpart may be successful with percent fat accumulations in the mid 20's. Studies vary but most authorities would argue that a male of 24 percent and a female of 30 percent fat are very near to obesity.

Skinfolds	Males (age in years)				Females (age in years)			
(mm)	17-29	30-39	40-49	50+	16-29	30-39	40-49	50+
20	8.1	12.2	12.2	12.6	14.1	17.0	19.8	21.4
25	10.5	14.2	15.0	15.6	16.8	19.4	22.2	24.0
30	12.9	16.2	17.7	18.6	19.5	21.8	24.5	26.6
35	14.7	17.7	19.6	20.8	21.5	23.7	26.4	28.5
40	16.4	19.2	21.4	22.9	23.4	25.5	28.2	30.3
45	17.7	20.4	23.0	24.7	25.0	26.9	29.6	31.9
50	19.0	21.5	24.6	26.5	26.5	28.2	31.0	33.4
55	20.1	22.5	25.9	27.9	27.8	29.4	32.1	34.6
60	21.2	23.5	27.1	29.2	29.1	30.6	33.2	35.7
65	22.2	24.3	28.2	30.4	30.2	31.6	34.1	36.7
70	23.1	25.1	29.3	31.6	31.2	32.5	35.0	37.7
75	24.0	25.9	30.3	32.7	32.2	33.4	35.9	38.7
80	24.8	26.6	31.2	33.8	33.1	34.3	36.7	39.6
85	25.5	27.2	32.1	34.8	34.0	35.1	37.5	40.4
90	26.2	27.8	33.0	35.8	34.8	35.8	38.3	41.2
95	26.9	28.4	33.7	36.6	35.6	36.5	39.0	41.9
100	27.6	29.0	34.4	37.4	36.4	37.2	39.7	42.6
105	28.2	29.6	35.1	38.2	37.1	37.9	40.4	43.3
110	28.8	30.1	35.8	39.0	37.8	38.6	41.0	43.9
115	29.4	30.6	36.4	39.7	38.4	39.1	41.5	44.5
120	30.0	31.1	37.0	40.4	39.0	39.6	42.0	45.1
125	30.5	31.5	37.6	41.1	39.6	40.1	42.5	45.7
130	31.0	31.9	38.2	41.8	40.2	40.6	43.0	46.2
135	31.5	32.3	38.7	42.4	40.8	41.1	43.5	46.7
140	32.0	32.7	39.2	43.0	41.3	41.6	44.0	47.2
145	32.5	33.1	39.7	43.6	41.8	42.1	44.5	47.7
150	32.9	33.5	40.2	44.1	42.3	42.6	45.0	48.2
155	33.3	33.9	40.7	44.6	42.8	43.1	45.4	48.7
160	33.7	34.3	41.2	45.1	43.3	43.6	45.8	49.2
165	34.1	34.6	41.6	45.6	43.7	44.0	46.2	49.6
170	34.5	34.8	42.0	46.1	44.1	44.4	46.6	50.0

APPENDIX B

Calorie expenditure for various types of physical activity. These are approximate values with variation due to skill and level of competition (vigour of play). You should add 10 per cent for every fifteen pounds of weight over 150 pounds. If you weigh less than 150 pounds, you should subtract 10 per cent for each 15 pounds.

Activity	Calorie expenditure per minute
Aerobic dance	6-9
Archery	5
Backpacking	6-14
Badminton	5-11
Basketball	
1/2 court	6-9
game play – full court	8-12
Bowling	5-6
Baseball (except pitcher)	5-6
Canoeing, rowing or kayaking	3-8
Calisthenics	5
Chopping wood	7-8
Cycling 5-15 mph (10 speed)	5-12
Carpentry	3-9
Dancing:	
disco	7-9
modern	4-6
social and square	4-7
Driving a Car	3
Dressing	3.5
Driving a motorcycle	3.5

Activity	Calorie expenditure per minute
Driving a heavy truck	4.0
Farming, ploughing with horse, haymaking	6-7
Fishing:	
from bank, boat or ice	3-5
stream, wading	7-8
Football (American) — touch	8-10
Football (soccer)	8-12
Gardening (digging, etc.)	8-9
Golf:	
power cart	3
walking (carrying bag or pulling cart)	3-6
Handball and squash	8-12
Horseback riding	3-10
Horseshoe pitching	4
Hunting (bow or gun)	5-9
Hunting (big game, dragging carcass, walking)	5-17
Home improvement (painting, plumbing, etc.)	4-5
Heavy housework (scrubbing floors, etc.)	5-6
Heavy tools:	
pneumatic tools, jackhammer	4-6
pick, shovel, etc.	6-7
Jogging	See Table 5.3, p. 00
Ironing clothes	4
Lifting and carrying objects:	
20-44 lb.	5.5
45-64 lb.	7.5
65-84 lb.	9.0
85-100 lb.	10.5
Judo and karate	8-12
Light housework (sweeping, polishing, etc.)	3-4
Lying quietly in bed	1.3
Mountain climbing	10-12
Paddleball or racquetball	8-12
Pool or billiards	2.0
Ping-pong — table tennis	5-9
Sailing	3-7
Scuba diving	7-13
Shuffleboard	3-4
Skating, ice or roller	5-15
Skiing, snow:	
downhill	8-12
cross-country	9-17

Activity	Calorie expenditure per minute
Sexual intercourse	4-6
Skiing, water	8
Standing (bartending)	2-3
Sledging (and tobogganing)	5-10
Snowshoeing (2.5 mph)	9.0
Squash and handball	8-12
Softball	5-6
Sitting	1.5
Showering	3.5
Stone, masonry	6-7
Shovelling snow:	
wet snow	10-17
powder snow	8-12
Skipping with rope	8-11
Swimming:	
crawl: 25-50 yd./min.	6-12
butterfly: 50 yd./min.	14
backstroke: 25-50 yd./min.	6-12.5
breaststroke: 25-50 yd./min.	6-12.5
sidestroke: 40 yd./min.	11.0
Tennis	7-12
Volleyball	4-8
Walking	See Table 5.3, p. 66

CALORIE, PROTEIN, FAT AND CARBOHYDRATE PARTS OF FOOD

Food, approximate measure, and weight (in grams)	Calories	Protein	Fat	Carbo-hydrate
MILK, CHEESE, CREAM, IMITATION CREAM; RELATED PRODUCTS	*Grams*	*Grams*	*Grams*	*Grams* *Grams*

Milk:
  Fluid:

		Grams	Calories	Protein	Fat	Carbo.
1	Whole, 3.5% fat . . . . . .1 cup	244	160	9	9	12
2	Nonfat (skim) . . . . . . .1 cup	245	90	9	Trace	12
3	Partly skimmed, 2%. . . .1 cup . . . . nonfat milk solids added.	246	145	10	5	15

  Canned, concentrated, undiluted:

4	Evaporated, un-sweetened.	1 cup	252	345	18	20	24
5	Condensed, sweetened.	1 cup	306	980	25	27	166

  Dry, nonfat instant:

6	Low-density (1⅓ cups needed for recon-stitution to 1 qt.).	1 cup	68	245	24	Trace	35
7	High-density (⅞ cup needed for recon-stitution to 1 qt.).	1 cup	104	375	37	1	54

  Buttermilk:

8	Fluid, cultured, made from skim milk.	1 cup	245	90	9	Trace	12
9	Dried, packaged . . . . . .1 cup		120	465	41	6	60

Cheese:
  Natural:
    Blue or Roquefort type:

10	Ounce . . . . .1 oz.		28	105	6	9	1
11	Cubic inch . . . . .1 cu. in		17	65	4	5	Trace

Food, approximate measure, and weight (in grams)			Calorie	Protein	Fat	Carbo-hydrate
MILK, CHEESE, CREAM, IMITATION CREAM; RELATED PRODUCTS		*Grams*	*Grams*	*Grams*	*Grams*	*Grams*
12	Camembert, packaged in 4-oz pkg. with 3 wedges per pkg.	1 wedge 38	115	7	9	1
	Cheddar:					
13	Ounce . . . . .1 oz.	28	115	7	9	1
14	Cubic inch . . . . .1 cu in	17	70	4	6	Trace
	Cottage, large or small curd:					
	Creamed:					
15	Package of 12-oz., net wt.	1 pkg 340	360	46	14	10
16	Cup, curd pressed down.	1 cup 245	260	33	10	7
	Uncreamed:					
17	Package of 12-oz., net wt.	1 pkg 340	290	58	1	9
18	Cup, curd pressed down.	1 cup 200	170	34	1	5
	Cream:					
19	Package of 8-oz., net wt.	1 pkg 227	850	18	86	5
20	Package of 3-oz., net wt.	1 pkg 85	320	7	32	2
21	Cubic inch . . . . .1 cu. in.	16	60	1	6	Trace
	Parmesan, grated:					
22	Cup, pressed down. . . .1 cup	140	655	60	43	5
23	Tablespoon . . . . . . .1 tbsp.	5	25	2	2	Trace
24	Ounce . . . . .1 oz.	28	130	12	9	1
	Swiss:					
25	Ounce . . . . .1 oz.	28	105	8	8	1
26	Cubic inch . . . . .1 cu. in.	15	55	4	4	Trace
	American:					
27	Ounce . . . . .1 oz.	28	105	7	9	1
28	Cubic inch . . . . .1 cu. in.	18	65	4	5	Trace
	Swiss:					
29	Ounce . . . . .1 oz.	28	100	8	8	1
30	Cubic inch . . . . .1 cu. in.	18	65	5	5	Trace
	Pasteurized process cheese food, American:					
31	Tablespoon . . . . . . .1 tbsp.	14	45	3	3	1
32	Cubic inch . . . . .1 cu. in.	18	60	4	4	1
33	Pasteurized process cheese spread, American.	1 oz. 28	80	5	6	2
	Cream:					
34	Half-and-half (cream and milk).	1 cup 242	325	8	28	11
35		1 tbsp. 15	20	1	2	1
36	Light, coffee or table . . .1 cup	240	505	7	49	10

	Food, approximate measure, and weight (in grams)			Calorie	Protein	Fat	Carbo-hydrate

MILK, CHEESE, CREAM, IMITATION CREAM; RELATED PRODUCTS

			Grams	Grams	Grams	Grams	Grams
37		1 tbsp.	15	30	1	3	1
38	Sour	1 cup	230	485	7	47	10
39		1 tbsp.	12	25	Trace	2	1
40	Whipped topping (pressurized).	1 cup	60	155	2	14	6
41		1 tbsp.	3	10	Trace	1	Trace
	Whipping, unwhipped (volume about double when whipped):						
42	Light	1 cup	239	715	6	75	9
43		1 tbsp.	15	45	Trace	5	1
44	Heavy.	1 cup	238	840	5	90	7
45		1 tbsp.	15	55	Trace	6	1
	Imitation cream products (made with vegetable fat): Creamers:						
46	Powdered	1 cup	94	505	4	33	52
47		1 tsp	2	10	Trace	1	1
48	Liquid (frozen)	1 cup	245	345	3	27	25
49		1 tbsp.	15	20	Trace	2	2
50	Sour dressing (imitation sour cream) made with nonfat dry milk.	1 cup	235	440	9	38	17
51		1 tbsp.	12	20	Trace	2	1
	Whipped topping:						
52	Pressurized.	1 cup	70	190	1	17	9
53		1 tbsp.	4	10	Trace	1	Trace
54	Frozen	1 cup	75	230	1	20	15
55		1 tbsp.	4	10	Trace	1	1
56	Powdered, made with whole milk.	1 cup	75	175	3	12	15
57		1 tbsp.	4	10	Trace	1	1
	Milk beverages:						
58	Cocoa, homemade	1 cup	250	245	10	12	27
59	Chocolate-flavored drink made with skim milk and 2% added butterfat.	1 cup	250	190	8	6	27
	Malted milk:						
60	Dry powder, approx. 3 heaping teaspoons per ounce.	1 oz.	28	115	4	2	20
61	Beverage	1 cup	235	245	11	10	28
	Milk desserts:						
62	Custard, baked	1 cup	265	305	14	15	29
	Ice cream:						
63	Regular (approx. 10% fat).	½ gal	1,064	2,055	48	113	221
64		1 cup	133	255	6	14	28
65		3 fl. oz. cup . . .	50	95	2	5	10

Food, approximate measure, and weight (in grams)		Calorie	Protein	Fat	Carbo-hydrate
MILK, CHEESE, CREAM, IMITATION CREAM; RELATED PRODUCTS	*Grams*	*Grams*	*Grams*	*Grams*	*Grams*
66	Rich (approx. 16% fat). ½ gal 1,188	2,635	31	191	214
67	1 cup 148	330	4	24	27
	Ice milk:				
68	Hardened. . . . . .½ gal 1,048	1,595	50	53	235
69	1 cup 131	200	6	7	29
70	Soft-serve . . . . .1 cup 175	265	8	9	39
	Yoghurt:				
71	Made from partially skimmed milk. 1 cup 245	125	8	4	13
72	Made from whole milk. 1 cup 245	150	7	8	12
	EGGS				
	Eggs, large, 24 ounces per dozen:				
	Raw or cooked in shell or with nothing added:				
73	Whole, without shell . . .1 egg	50	80	6	6	Trace
74	White of egg . . . . .1 white.	33	15	4	Trace	Trace
75	Yolk of egg . . . . . . .1 yolk	17	60	3	5	Trace
76	Scrambled with milk and fat. 1 egg	64	110	7	8	1
	MEAT, POULTRY, FISH, SHELLFISH; RELATED PRODUCTS				
77	Bacon (20 slices per lb. raw), broiled or fried, crisp. 2 slices	15	90	5	8	1
	Beef, cooked:				
	Cuts braised, simmered, or pot-roasted:				
78	Lean and fat. . . . . . . .3 ounces	85	245	23	16	0
79	Lean only . . . . .2.5 ounces	72	140	22	5	0
	Hamburger (ground beef), broiled:				
80	Lean . . . . .3 ounces	85	185	23	10	0
81	Regular. . . . . .3 ounces	85	245	21	17	0
	Roast, oven-cooked, no liquid added:				
	Relatively fat, such as rib:				
82	Lean and fat. . . . . . .3 ounces	85	375	17	34	0
83	Lean only . . . . .1.8 ounces	51	125	14	7	0
	Relatively lean, such as heel of round:				
84	Lean and fat. . . . . . .3 ounces	85	165	25	7	0
85	Lean only . . . . .2.7 ounces	78	125	24	3	0
	Steak, broiled:				
	Relatively fat, such as sirloin:				
86	Lean and fat. . . . . . .3 ounces	85	330	20	27	0
87	Lean only . . . . .2.0 ounces	56	115	18	4	0
	Relatively lean, such as round:				
88	Lean and fat. . . . . . .3 ounces	85	220	24	13	0
89	Lean only . . . . .2.4 ounces	68	130	21	4	0

Food, approximate measure, and weight (in grams)			Calorie	Protein	Fat	Carbo-hydrate
MEAT, POULTRY, FISH, SHELLFISH; RELATED PRODUCTS		*Grams*	*Grams*	*Grams*	*Grams*	*Grams*
	Beef, canned:					
90	Corned beef . . . . .3 ounces	85	185	22	10	0
91	Corned beef hash . . . . . .3 ounces	85	155	7	10	9
92	Beef, dried or chipped . . . .2 ounces	57	115	19	4	0
93	Beef and vegetable stew . . .1 cup	235	210	15	10	15
94	Beef potpie, baked, 4¼- 1 pie . . . . inch diam., weight before baking about 8 ounces.	227	560	23	33	43
	Chicken, cooked:					
95	Flesh only, broiled . . . . .3 ounces	85	115	20	3	0
	Breast, fried, ½ breast:					
96	With bone . . . . .3.3 ounces	94	155	25	5	1
97	Flesh and skin only . . . .2.7 ounces	76	155	25	5	1
	Drumstick, fried:					
98	With bone . . . . .2.1 ounces	59	90	12	4	Trace
99	Flesh and skin only . . . .1.3 ounces	38	90	12	4	Trace
100	Chicken, canned, boneless . .3 ounces	85	170	18	10	0
101	Chicken, potpie, baked 4¼- 1 pie . . . . inch diam., weight before baking about 8 ounces.	227	535	23	31	42
	Chili con carne, canned:					
102	With beans . . . . .1 cup	250	335	19	15	30
103	Without beans . . . . .1 cup	255	510	26	38	15
104	Heart, beef, lean, braised. . .3 ounces	85	160	27	5	1
	Lamb, cooked:					
105	Chop, thick, with bone. . .1 chop . . . . . . broiled. 4.8 ounces	137	400	25	33	0
106	Lean and fat . . . . . . .4.0 ounces	112	400	25	33	0
107	Lean only . . . . .2.6 ounces	74	140	21	6	0
	Leg, roasted:					
108	Lean and fat . . . . . . .3 ounces	85	235	22	16	0
109	Lean only . . . . .2.5 ounces	71	130	20	5	0
	Shoulder, roasted:					
110	Lean and fat . . . . . . .3 ounces	85	285	18	23	0
111	Lean only . . . . .2.3 ounces	64	130	17	6	0
112	Liver, beef, fried . . . . . . .2 ounces	57	130	15	6	3
	Pork, cured, cooked:					
113	Ham, light cure, lean and 3 ounces . . . . . fat, roasted.	85	245	18	19	0
	Luncheon meat:					
114	Boiled ham, sliced. . . . .2 ounces	57	135	11	10	0
115	Canned, spiced or 2 ounces . . . . . unspiced.	57	165	8	14	1
	Pork, fresh, cooked:					
116	Chop, thick, with bone. . .1 chop, 3.5 ounces.	98	260	16	21	0
117	Lean and fat . . . . . . .2.3 ounces	66	260	16	21	0
118	Lean only . . . . .1.7 ounces	48	130	15	7	0

Food, approximate measure, and weight (in grams)			Calorie	Protein	Fat	Carbo-hydrate
MEAT, POULTRY, FISH, SHELLFISH; RELATED PRODUCTS		*Grams*	*Grams*	*Grams*	*Grams*	*Grams*
	Roast, oven-cooked, no liquid added:					
119	Lean and fat . . . . . . .3 ounces	85	310	21	24	0
120	Lean only . . . . .2.4 ounces	68	175	20	10	0
	Cuts, simmered:					
121	Lean and fat . . . . . . .3 ounces	85	320	20	26	0
122	Lean only . . . . .2.2 ounces	63	135	18	6	0
	Sausage:					
123	Bologna, slice, 3-in. diam. 2 slices . . . . . . by ⅛ inch.	26	80	3	7	Trace
124	Braunschweiger, slice 2 slices . . . . . . 2-in. diam. by ¼ inch.	20	65	3	5	Trace
125	Deviled ham, canned . . . .1 tbsp.	13	45	2	4	0
126	Frankfurter, heated (8 1 frank . . . . . . per lb. purchased pkg.).	56	170	7	15	1
127	Pork links, cooked (16 2 links . . . . . . links per lb. raw).	26	125	5	11	Trace
128	Salami, dry type. . . . . . .1 oz.	28	130	7	11	Trace
129	Salami, cooked . . . . . . .1 oz.	28	90	5	7	Trace
130	Vienna, canned (7 1 sausage . . . . . sausages per 5-oz. can.).	16	40	2	3	Trace
	Veal, medium fat, cooked, bone removed:					
131	Cutlet. . . . . .3 oz.	85	185	23	9	0
132	Roast . . . . .3 oz.	85	230	23	14	0
	Fish and shellfish:					
133	Bluefish, baked with 3 oz. . . . . table fat.	85	135	22	4	0
	Clams:					
134	Raw, meat only . . . . .3 oz.	85	65	11	1	2
135	Canned, solids and 3 oz. . . . . .liquid.	85	45	7	1	2
136	Crabmeat, canned. . . . .3 oz.	85	85	15	2	1
137	Fish sticks, breaded, 10 sticks or cooked, frozen: stick 8 oz. pkg. 3¾ by 1 by ½ inch.	227	400	38	20	15
138	Haddock, breaded, fried . .3 oz.	85	140	17	5	5
139	Ocean perch, breaded, 3 oz. . . . . fried.	85	195	16	11	6
140	Oysters, raw, meat only 1 cup . . . . (13-19 med. selects).	240	160	20	4	8
141	Salmon, pink, canned. . . .3 oz.	85	120	17	5	0
142	Sardines, Atlantic, canned 3 oz. . . . . in oil, drained solids.	85	175	20	9	0
143	Shad, baked with table 3 oz. . . . . fat and bacon.	85	170	20	10	0
144	Shrimp, canned, meat . . .3 oz.	85	100	21	1	1
145	Swordfish, broiled with 3 oz. . . . . butter or margarine.	85	150	24	5	0

	Food, approximate measure, and weight (in grams)		Calorie	Protein	Fat	Carbo-hydrate
	MEAT, POULTRY, FISH, SHELLFISH; RELATED PRODUCTS	*Grams*	*Grams*	*Grams*	*Grams*	*Grams*
146	Tuna, canned in oil, drained solids.	3 oz. 85	170	24	7	0
	MATURE DRY BEANS AND PEAS, NUTS, PEANUTS; RELATED PRODUCTS					
147	Almonds, shelled, whole kernels.	1 cup 142	850	26	77	28
	Beans, dry:					
	Common varieties as Great Northern, navy, and others:					
	Cooked, drained:					
148	Great Northern	1 cup 180	210	14	1	38
149	Navy (pea).	1 cup 190	225	15	1	40
	Canned, solids and liquid:					
	White with—					
150	Frankfurters (sliced)	.1 cup 255	365	19	18	32
151	Pork and tomato sauce.	1 cup 255	310	16	7	49
152	Pork and sweet sauce.	1 cup 255	385	16	12	54
153	Red kidney	1 cup 255	230	15	1	42
154	Lima, cooked, drained . .	.1 cup 190	260	16	1	49
155	Cashew nuts, roasted	.1 cup 140	785	24	64	41
	Coconut, fresh, meat only:					
156	Pieces, approx. 2 by 2 by ½ inch.	1 piece 45	155	2	16	4
157	Shredded or grated, firmly packed.	1 cup 130	450	5	46	12
158	Cowpeas or blackeye peas, dry, cooked.	1 cup 248	190	13	1	34
159	Peanuts, roasted, salted	1 cup 144	840	37	72	27
160	Peanut butter	.1 tbsp. 16	95	4	8	3
161	Peas, split, dry, cooked. . . .	.1 cup 250	290	20	1	52
162	Pecans, halves	.1 cup 108	740	10	77	16
163	Walnuts, black or native, chopped.	1 cup 126	790	26	75	19
	VEGETABLES AND VEGETABLE PRODUCTS					
	Asparagus, green:					
	Cooked, drained:					
164	Spears, ½-in. diam. at base.	4 spears. 60	10	1	Trace	2
165	Pieces, 1½ to 2-in. lengths.	1 cup 145	30	3	Trace	5

140

Food, approximate measure, and weight (in grams)			Calorie	Protein	Fat	Carbo-hydrate
VEGETABLES AND VEGETABLE PRODUCTS		*Grams*	*Grams*	*Grams*	*Grams*	*Grams*
166	Canned, solids and liquid.	1 cup 244	45	5	1	7
	Beans:					
167	Lima, immature seeds, cooked, drained.	1 cup 170	190	13	1	34
	Snap:					
	Green:					
168	Cooked, drained. . . . .1 cup 125		30	2	Trace	7
169	Canned, solids and liquid.	1 cup 239	45	2	Trace	10
	Yellow or wax:					
170	Cooked, drained. . . . .1 cup 125		30	2	Trace	6
171	Canned, solids and liquid.	1 cup 239	45	2	1	10
172	Sprouted mung beans, cooked, drained.	1 cup 125	35	4	Trace	7
	Beets:					
	Cooked, drained, peeled:					
173	Whole beets, 2-in. diam. .2 beets 100		30	1	Trace	7
174	Diced or sliced. . . . . . .1 cup 170		55	2	Trace	12
175	Canned, solids and liquid. .1 cup 246		85	2	Trace	19
176	Beet greens, leaves and stems, cooked, drained.	1 cup 145	25	3	Trace	5
	Blackeye peas. See Cowpeas.					
	Broccoli, cooked, drained:					
177	Whole stalks, medium size.	1 stalk 180	45	6	1	8
178	Stalks cut into ½-in. pieces.	1 cup 155	40	5	1	7
179	Chopped, yield from 10-oz. frozen pkg.	1⅜ cups 250	65	7	1	12
180	Brussels sprouts, 7-8 sprouts (1¼ to 1½ in. diam.) per cup, cooked.	1 cup 155	55	7	1	10
	Cabbage:					
	Common varieties:					
	Raw:					
181	Coarsely shredded or sliced.	1 cup 70	15	1	Trace	4
182	Finely shredded or chopped.	1 cup 90	20	1	Trace	5
183	Cooked. . . . . .1 cup 145		30	2	Trace	6
184	Red, raw, coarsely shredded.	1 cup 70	20	1	Trace	5
185	Savoy, raw, coarsely shredded.	1 cup 70	15	2	Trace	3
186	Cabbage, celery or Chinese, raw, cut in 1-in. pieces.	1 cup 75	10	1	Trace	2

Food, approximate measure, and weight (in grams)		Calorie	Protein	Fat	Carbo-hydrate
VEGETABLES AND VEGETABLE PRODUCTS		*Grams*	*Grams*	*Grams*	*Grams* *Grams*
187 Cabbage, spoon (or pakchoy), cooked.	1 cup 170	25	2	Trace	4
Carrots: Raw:					
188 Whole, 5½ by 1 inch, (25 thin strips).	1 carrot. 50	20	1	Trace	5
189 Grated	.1 cup 110	45	1	Trace	11
190 Cooked, diced	.1 cup 145	45	1	Trace	10
191 Canned, strained or chopped (baby food).	1 ounce. 28	10	Trace	Trace	2
192 Cauliflower, cooked, flowerbuds.	1 cup 120	25	3	Trace	5
Celery, raw:					
193 Stalk, large outer, 8 by about 1½ inches, at root end.	1 stalk 40	5	Trace	Trace	2
194 Pieces, diced	.1 cup 100	15	1	Trace	4
195 Collards, cooked	.1 cup 190	55	5	1	9
Corn, sweet:					
196 Cooked, ear 5 by 1¾ inches.	1 ear 140	70	3	1	16
197 Canned, solids and liquid.	.1 cup 256	170	5	2	40
198 Cowpeas, cooked, immature seeds.	1 cup 160	175	13	1	29
Cucumbers, 10-ounce; 7½ by about 2 inches:					
199 Raw, pared.	.1 cucumber . . . 207	30	1	Trace	7
200 Raw, pared, center slice ⅛ -inch thick.	6 slices 50	5	Trace	Trace	2
201 Dandelion greens, cooked .	.1 cup 180	60	4	1	12
202 Endive, curly (including escarole).	2 ounces 57	10	1	Trace	2
203 Kale, leaves including stems, cooked.	1 cup 110	30	4	1	4
Lettuce, raw:					
204 Butterhead, as Boston types; head, 4-inch diameter.	1 head 220	30	3	Trace	6
205 Crisphead, as Iceberg; head, 4¾-inch diameter.	1 head 454	60	4	Trace	13
206 Looseleaf, or bunching varieties, leaves.	2 large 50	10	1	Trace	2
207 Mushrooms, canned, solids and liquid.	1 cup 244	40	5	Trace	6
208 Mustard greens, cooked . .	.1 cup 140	35	3	1	6
209 Okra, cooked, pod 3 by ⅝ inch.	8 pods 85	25	2	Trace	5

	Food, approximate measure, and weight (in grams)		Calorie	Protein	Fat	Carbo-hydrate
	VEGETABLES AND VEGETABLE PRODUCTS		*Grams*	*Grams*	*Grams*	*Grams* *Grams*
	Onions:					
	Mature:					
210	Raw, onion 2½-inch diameter.	1 onion 110	40	2	Trace	10
211	Cooked . . . . .1 cup 210		60	3	Trace	14
212	Young green, small, without tops.	6 onions 50	20	1	Trace	5
213	Parsley, raw, chopped . . . .1 tablespoon. . . 4		Trace	Trace	Trace	Trace
214	Parsnips, cooked . . . . . . .1 cup 155		100	2	1	23
	Peas, green:					
215	Cooked . . . . .1 cup 160		115	9	1	19
216	Canned, solids and liquid. .1 cup 249		165	9	1	31
217	Canned, strained (baby food).	1 ounce 28	15	1	Trace	3
218	Peppers, hot, red, without seeds, dried (ground chili powder, added seasonings).	1 tablespoon. . . 15	50	2	2	8
	Peppers, sweet:					
	Raw, about 5 per pound:					
219	Green pod without stem and seeds.	1 pod 74	15	1	Trace	4
220	Cooked, boiled, drained . .1 pod 73		15	1	Trace	3
	Potatoes, medium (about 3 per pound raw):					
221	Baked, peeled after baking.	1 potato 99	90	3	Trace	21
	Boiled:					
222	Peeled after boiling . . . .1 potato 136		105	3	Trace	23
223	Peeled before boiling . . .1 potato 122		80	2	Trace	18
	French-fried, piece 2 by ½ by ½ inch:					
224	Cooked in deep fat . . . .10 pieces. 57		155	2	7	20
225	Frozen, heated . . . . . .10 pieces. 57		125	2	5	19
	Mashed:					
226	Milk added . . . . .1 cup 195		125	4	1	25
227	Milk and butter added . .1 cup 195		185	4	8	24
228	Potato chips, medium, 2-inch diameter.	10 chips 20	115	1	8	10
229	Pumpkin, canned . . . . . .1 cup 228		75	2	1	18
230	Radishes, raw, small, without tops.	4 radishes 40	5	Trace	Trace	1
231	Sauerkraut, canned, solids and liquids.	1 cup 235	45	2	Trace	9
	Spinach:					
232	Cooked . . . . .1 cup 180		40	5	1	6
233	Canned, drained solids . . .1 cup 180		45	5	1	6
	Squash:					
	Cooked:					
234	Summer, diced . . . . . .1 cup 210		30	2	Trace	7

Food, approximate measure, and weight (in grams)		Calorie	Protein	Fat	Carbo-hydrate

VEGETABLES AND VEGETABLE PRODUCTS

		Grams	Grams	Grams	Grams	Grams
235	Winter, baked, mashed . .1 cup	205	130	4	1	32
	Sweetpotatoes:					
	Cooked, medium, 5 by 2 inches, weight raw about 6 ounces:					
236	Baked, peeled after . . . .1 sweetpotato . .	110	155	2	1	36
	baking.					
237	Boiled, peeled after 1 sweetpotato . .	147	170	2	1	39
	boiling.					
238	Candied, 3½ by 2¼ 1 sweetpotato . .	175	295	2	6	60
	inches.					
239	Canned, vacuum or 1 cup	218	235	4	Trace	54
	solid pack.					
	Tomatoes:					
240	Raw, approx. 3-in. diam. 1 tomato	200	40	2	Trace	9
	2⅛ in. high; wt., 7 oz.					
241	Canned, solids and liquid. .1 cup	241	50	2	1	10
	Tomato catsup:					
242	Cup . . . . .1 cup	273	290	6	1	69
243	Tablespoon . . . . .1 tbsp.	15	15	Trace	Trace	4
	Tomato juice, canned:					
244	Cup . . . . .1 cup	243	45	2	Trace	10
245	Glass (6 fl. oz.) . . . . . . .1 glass	182	35	2	Trace	8
246	Turnips, cooked, diced . . . .1 cup	155	35	1	Trace	8
247	Turnip greens, cooked . . . .1 cup	145	30	3	Trace	5

FRUITS AND FRUIT PRODUCTS

		Grams	Grams	Grams	Grams	Grams
248	Apples, raw (about 3 1 apple	150	70	Trace	Trace	18
	per lb.).					
249	Apple juice, bottled or 1 cup	248	120	Trace	Trace	30
	canned.					
	Applesauce, canned:					
250	Sweetened . . . . .1 cup	255	230	1	Trace	61
251	Unsweetened or artifi- 1 cup	244	100	1	Trace	26
	cially sweetened.					
	Apricots:					
252	Raw (about 12 per lb.) . .3 apricots	114	55	1	Trace	14
253	Canned in heavy sirup . . .1 cup	259	220	2	Trace	57
254	Dried, uncooked (40 1 cup	150	390	8	1	100
	halves per cup).					
255	Cooked, unsweetened, 1 cup	285	240	5	1	62
	fruit and liquid.					
256	Apricot nectar, canned . . . .1 cup	251	140	1	Trace	37
	Avocados, whole fruit, raw:					
257	California (mid- and late- 1 avocado	284	370	5	37	13
	winter; diam. 3⅛ in.).					

Food, approximate measure, and weight (in grams)			Calorie	Protein	Fat	Carbo-hydrate
FRUITS AND FRUIT PRODUCTS		*Grams*	*Grams*	*Grams*	*Grams*	*Grams*
258	Florida (late summer, fall; diam. 3⅝ in.).	1 avocado 454	390	4	33	27
259	Bananas, raw, medium size.	.1 banana 175	100	1	Trace	26
260	Banana flakes	.1 cup 100	340	4	1	89
261	Blackberries, raw	.1 cup 144	85	2	1	19
262	Blueberries, raw	.1 cup 140	85	1	1	21
263	Cantaloups, raw; medium; 5-inch diameter about 1⅔ pounds.	½ melon 385	60	1	Trace	14
264	Cherries, canned, red, sour, pitted, water pack.	1 cup 244	105	2	Trace	26
265	Cranberry juice cocktail, canned.	1 cup 250	165	Trace	Trace	42
266	Cranberry sauce, sweetened, canned, strained.	1 cup 277	330	Trace	1	85
267	Dates, pitted, cut	.1 cup 178	490	4	1	130
268	Figs, dried, large, 2 by 1 in.	.1 fig. 21	60	1	Trace	15
269	Fruit cocktail, canned, in heavy sirup.	1 cup 256	195	1	Trace	50
	Grapefruit: Raw, medium, 3¾-in. diam.					
270	White	.½ grapefruit . . . 241	45	1	Trace	12
271	Pink or red	.½ grapefruit . . . 241	50	1	Trace	13
272	Canned, sirup pack	.1 cup 254	180	2	Trace	45
	Grapefruit juice:					
273	Fresh	.1 cup 246	95	1	Trace	23
	Canned, white:					
274	Unsweetened	.1 cup 247	100	1	Trace	24
275	Sweetened	.1 cup 250	130	1	Trace	32
	Frozen, concentrate, unsweetened:					
276	Undiluted, can, 6 fluid ounces.	1 can 207	300	4	1	72
277	Diluted with 3 parts water, by volume.	1 cup 247	100	1	Trace	24
278	Dehydrated crystals. . .	.4 oz. 113	410	6	1	102
279	Prepared with water (1 pound yields about 1 gallon).	1 cup 247	100	1	Trace	24
	Grapes, raw:					
280	American type (slip skin) .	1 cup 153	65	1	1	15
281	European type (adherent skin).	1 cup 160	95	1	Trace	25
	Grapejuice:					
282	Canned or bottled	.1 cup 253	165	1	Trace	42
	Frozen concentrate, sweetened:					
283	Undiluted, can, 6 fluid ounces.	1 can 216	395	1	Trace	100

Food, approximate measure, and weight (in grams)			Calorie	Protein	Fat	Carbo-hydrate

	FRUITS AND FRUIT PRODUCTS		*Grams*	*Grams*	*Grams*	*Grams*	*Grams*
284	Diluted with 3 parts water, by volume.	1 cup 250	135	1	Trace	33
285	Grapejuice drink, canned. . .	1 cup 250	135	Trace	Trace	35
286	Lemons, raw, 2⅛-in. diameter zie 165. Used for juice.	1 lemon 110	20	1	Trace	6
287	Lemon juice, raw	1 cup 244	60	1	Trace	20
	Lemonade concentrate:					
288	Frozen, 6 fl. oz. per can . .	1 can 219	430	Trace	Trace	112
289	Diluted with 4⅓ parts water, by volume.	1 cup 248	110	Trace	Trace	28
	Lime juice:					
290	Fresh	1 cup 246	65	1	Trace	22
291	Canned, unsweetened. . . .	1 cup 246	65	1	Trace	22
	Limeade concentrate, frozen:					
292	Undiluted, can, 6 fluid ounces.	1 can 218	410	Trace	Trace	108
293	Diluted with 4⅓ parts water, by volume.	1 cup 247	100	Trace	Trace	27
294	Oranges, raw, 2⅝-in. diam., all commercial varieties.	1 orange 180	65	1	Trace	16
295	Orange juice, fresh, all varieties.	1 cup 248	110	2	1	26
296	Canned, unsweetened. . . .	1 cup 249	120	2	Trace	28
	Frozen concentrate:					
297	Undiluted, can, 6 fluid ounces.	1 can 213	360	5	Trace	87
298	Diluted with 3 parts water, by volume.	1 cup 249	120	2	Trace	29
299	Dehydrated crystals. . . .	4 oz. 113	430	6	2	100
300	Prepared with water (1 pound yields about 1 gallon).	1 cup 248	115	2	1	27
301	Orange-apricot juice drink . .	1 cup 249	125	1	Trace	32
	Orange and grapefruit juice: Frozen concentrate:					
302	Undiluted, can, 6 fluid ounces.	1 can 210	330	4	1	78
303	Diluted with 3 parts water, by volume.	1 cup 248	110	1	Trace	26
304	Papayas, raw, ½-inch cubes .	1 cup 182	70	1	Trace	18
	Peaches: Raw:					
305	Whole, medium, 2-inch diameter, about 4 per pound.'	1 peach. 114	35	1	Trace	10
306	Sliced.	1 cup 168	65	1	Trace	16

Food, approximate measure, and weight (in grams)			Calorie	Protein	Fat	Carbo-hydrate
FRUITS AND FRUIT PRODUCTS		*Grams*	*Grams*	*Grams*	*Grams*	*Grams*
	Canned, yellow-fleshed, solids and liquid:					
	Sirup pack, heavy:					
307	Halves or slices . . . . .1 cup	257	200	1	Trace	52
308	Water pack. . . . . .1 cup	245	75	1	Trace	20
309	Dried, uncooked . . . . . .1 cup	160	420	5	1	109
310	Cooked, unsweetened, 1 cup . . . . . . 10-12 halves and juice.	270	220	3	1	58
	Frozen:					
311	Carton, 12 ounces, 1 carton . . . . . not thawed.	340	300	1	Trace	77
	Pears:					
312	Raw, 3 by 2½-inch 1 pear. . . . . . . diameter.	182	100	1	1	25
	Canned, solids and liquid:					
	Sirup pack, heavy:					
313	Halves or slices . . . . .1 cup	255	195	1	1	50
	Pineapple:					
314	Raw, diced. . . . . .1 cup	140	75	1	Trace	19
	Canned, heavy sirup pack, solids and liquid:					
315	Crushed . . . . .1 cup	260	195	1	Trace	50
316	Sliced, slices and juice . .2 small or 1 large.	122	90	Trace	Trace	24
317	Pineapple juice, canned. . . .1 cup	249	135	1	Trace	34
	Plums, all except prunces:					
318	Raw, 2-inch diameter, 1 plum . . . . . . about 2 ounces.	60	25	Trace	Trace	7
	Canned, sirup pack (Italian prunes):					
319	Plums (with pits) and 1 cup . . . . . . juice.	256	205	1	Trace	53
	Prunes, dried, "softenized", medium:					
320	Uncooked . . . . .4 prunes	32	70	1	Trace	18
321	Cooked, unsweetened, 1 cup . . . . . . 17-18 prunes and ⅓ cup liquid.	270	295	2	1	78
322	Prune juice, canned or 1 cup . . . . . . bottled.	256	200	1	Trace	49
	Raisins, seedless:					
323	Packaged, ½ oz. or 1½ 1 pkg . . . . . . tbsp. per pkg.	14	40	Trace	Trace	11
324	Cup, pressed down . . . . .1 cup	165	480	4	Trace	128
	Raspberries, red:					
325	Raw. . . . . .1 cup	123	70	1	1	17
326	Frozen, 10-ounce carton, 1 carton . . . . . not thawed.	284	275	2	1	70
327	Rhubarb, cooked, sugared 1 cup	272	385	1	Trace	98
	Strawberries:					
328	Raw, capped. . . . . . . .1 cup	149	55	1	1	13

147

Food, approximate measure, and weight (in grams)			Calorie	Protein	Fat	Carbo-hydrate
FRUITS AND FRUIT PRODUCTS		*Grams*	*Grams*	*Grams*	*Grams*	*Grams*
329 Frozen, 10-ounce carton, not thawed.	1 carton	284	310	1	1	79
330 Tangerines, raw, medium, 2⅜-in. diam. size 176.	1 tangerine. . . .	116	40	1	Trace	10
331 Tangerine juice, canned, sweetened.	1 cup	249	125	1	1	30
332 Watermelon, raw, wedge, 4 by 8 inches (¹⁄₁₆ of 10 by 16-inch melon, about 2 pounds with rind).	1 wedge	925	115	2	1	27
GRAIN PRODUCTS						
Bagel, 3-in. diam.:						
333 Egg	1 bagel	55	165	6	2	28
334 Water.	1 bagel	55	165	6	2	30
335 Barley, pearled, light, uncooked.	1 cup	200	700	16	2	158
336 Biscuits, baking powder from home recipe with enriched flour, 2-in. diam.	1 biscuit	28	105	2	5	13
337 Biscuits, baking powder from mix, 2-in. diam.	1 biscuit	28	90	2	3	15
338 Bran flakes (40% bran), added thiamin and iron.	1 cup	35	105	4	1	28
339 Bran flakes with raisins, added thiamin and iron.	1 cup	50	145	4	1	40
Breads:						
340 Boston brown bread, slice 3 by ¾ in.	1 slice.	48	100	3	1	22
Cracked-wheat bread:						
341 Loaf, 1 lb.	1 loaf.	454	1,190	40	10	236
342 Slice, 18 slices per loaf .	1 slice.	25	65	2	1	13
French or vienna bread:						
343 Enriched, 1 lb. loaf . . .	1 loaf.	454	1,315	41	14	251
344 Unenriched, 1 lb. loaf .	1 loaf.	454	1,315	41	14	251
Italian bread:						
345 Enriched, 1 lb. loaf . . .	1 loaf.	454	1,250	41	4	256
346 Unenriched, 1 lb. loaf .	1 loaf.	454	1,250	41	4	256
Raisin bread:						
347 Loaf, 1 lb.	1 loaf.	454	1,190	30	13	243
348 Slice, 18 slices per loaf .	1 slice.	25	65	2	1	13
Rye bread:						
American, light (⅓ rye, ⅔ wheat):						
349 Loaf, 1 lb	1 loaf.	454	1,100	41	5	236
350 Slice, 18 slices per loaf.	1 slice.	25	60	2	Trace	13

Food, approximate measure, and weight (in grams)		Calorie	Protein	Fat	Carbo-hydrate
GRAIN PRODUCTS	*Grams*	*Grams*	*Grams*	*Grams*	*Grams*
351 Pumpernickel, loaf, 1 lb . 1 loaf 454		1,115	41	5	241
White bread, enriched:					
Soft-crumb type:					
352 Loaf, 1 lb . . . . .1 loaf 454		1,225	39	15	229
353 Slice, 18 slices per loaf .1 slice 25		70	2	1	13
354 Slice, toasted . . . . .1 slice 22		70	2	1	13
355 Slice, 22 slices per loaf .1 slice 20		55	2	1	10
356 Slice, toasted . . . . .1 slice 17		55	2	1	10
357 Loaf, 1½ lbs . . . . . . .1 loaf 680		1,835	59	22	343
358 Slice, 24 slices per loaf .1 slice 28		75	2	1	14
359 Slice, toasted . . . . . .1 slice 24		75	2	1	14
360 Slice, 28 slices per loaf .1 slice 24		65	2	1	12
361 Slice, toasted . . . . . 1 slice 21		65	2	1	12
Firm-crumb type:					
362 Loaf, 1 lb . . . . .1 loaf 454		1,245	41	17	228
363 Slice, 20 slices per loaf .1 slice 23		65	2	1	12
364 Slice, toasted . . . . . .1 slice 20		65	2	1	12
365 Loaf, 2 lbs . . . . .1 loaf 907		2,495	82	34	455
366 Slice, 34 slices per loaf .1 slice 27		75	2	1	14
367 Slice toasted . . . . . .1 slice 23		75	2	1	14
Whole-wheat bread, soft-crumb type:					
368 Loaf, 1 lb . . . . .1 loaf 454		1,095	41	12	224
369 Slice, 16 slices per loaf . .1 slice 28		65	3	1	14
370 Slice, toasted . . . . . .1 slice 24		65	3	1	14
Whole-wheat bread, firm-crumb type:					
371 Loaf, 1 lb . . . . .1 loaf 454		1,100	48	14	216
372 Slice, 18 slices per loaf . . .1 slice 25		60	3	1	12
373 Slice, toasted . . . . . . .1 slice 21		60	3	1	12
374 Breadcrumbs, dry, grated . .1 cup 100		390	13	5	73
375 Buckwheat flour, light 1 cup 98		340	6	1	78
376 Bulgur, canned, seasoned. . .1 cup 135		245	8	4	44
Cakes made from cake mixes:					
Angelfood:					
377 Whole cake . . . . .1 cake 635		1,645	36	1	377
378 Piece, ¹⁄₁₂ of 10-in . . . . . .1 piece 53		135	3	Trace	32
diam. cake.					
Cupcakes, small, 2½-in. diam:					
379 Without icing . . . . . . .1 cupcake 25		90	1	3	14
380 With chocolate icing . . .1 cupcake 36		130	2	5	21
Devil's food, 2-layer, with chocolate icing:					
381 Whole cake . . . . .1 cake 1,107		3,755	49	136	645
382 Piece, ¹⁄₁₆ of 9-in. 1 piece 69		235	3	9	40
diam. cake.					
383 Cupcake, small, 2½- 1 cupcake 35		120	2	4	20
in. diam.					
Gingerbread:					
384 Whole cake . . . . .1 cake 570		1,575	18	39	291

Food, approximate measure, and weight (in grams)			Calorie	Protein	Fat	Carbo-hydrate
GRAIN PRODUCTS		*Grams*	*Grams*	*Grams*	*Grams*	*Grams*
385	Piece, ⅑ of 8-in. square cake.	1 piece 63	175	2	4	32
	White, 2-layer, with chocolate icing:					
386	Whole cake. . . . . .1 cake 1,140		4,000	45	122	716
387	Piece, ¹/₁₆ of 9-in. diam. cake.	1 piece 71	250	3	8	45
	Cakes made from home recipes:[16]					
388	Boston cream pie; piece ¹/₁₂ of 8-in. diam.	1 piece 69	210	4	6	34
	Fruitcake, dark, made with enriched flour:					
389	Loaf, 1-lb. . . . . .1 loaf. 454		1,720	22	69	271
390	Slice, 1/30 of 8-in. loaf. .1 slice. 15		55	1	2	9
	Plain sheet cake:					
	Without icing:					
391	Whole cake. . . . . . . .1 cake 777		2,830	35	108	434
392	Piece, ⅑ of 9-in. square cake.	1 piece 86	315	4	12	48
393	With boiled white icing, piece, ⅑ of 9-in. square cake.	1 piece 114	400	4	12	71
	Pound:					
394	Loaf, 8½ by 3½ by 3in. 1 loaf. 514		2,430	29	152	242
395	Slice, ½-in. thick . . . .1 slice. 30		140	2	9	14
	Sponge:					
396	Whole cake. . . . . . . .1 cake 790		2,345	60	45	427
397	Piece, ¹/₁₂ of 10-in. diam. cake.	1 piece 66	195	5	4	36
	Yellow, 2-layer, without icing:					
398	Whole cake. . . . . . . .1 cake 870		3,160	39	111	506
399	Piece, ¹/₁₆ of 9-in diam. cake.	1 piece 54	200	2	7	32
	Yellow, 2-layer, with chocolate icing:					
400	Whole cake. . . . . . . .1 cake 1,203		4,390	51	156	727
401	Piece, ¹/₁₆ of 9-in. diam. cake.	1 piece 75	275	3	10	45
	Cookies:					
	Brownies with nuts:					
402	Made from home recipe with enriched flour.	1 brownie 20	95	1	6	10
403	Made from mix . . . . . .1 brownie 20		85	1	4	13
	Chocolate chip:					
404	Made from home recipe with enriched flour.	1 cookie 10	50	1	3	6
405	Commercial . . . . .1 cookie 10		50	1	2	7
406	Fig bars, commercial . . . .1 cookie 14		50	1	1	11
407	Sandwich, chocolate or vanilla, commercial.	1 cookie 10	50	1	2	7

Food, approximate measure, and weight (in grams)			Calorie	Protein	Fat	Carbo-hydrate
GRAIN PRODUCTS		*Grams*	*Grams*	*Grams*	*Grams*	*Grams*
	Cornflakes, added nutrients:					
408	Plain . . . . .1 cup	25	100	2	Trace	21
409	Sugar-covered . . . . .1 cup	40	155	2	Trace	36
	Corn (hominy) grits, degermed, cooked:					
410	Enriched . . . . .1 cup	245	125	3	Trace	27
411	Unenriched . . . . .1 cup	245	125	3	Trace	27
	Cornmeal:					
412	Whole-ground, unbolted, dry.	1 cup	122	435	11	5	90
413	Bolted (nearly whole-grain) dry.	1 cup	122	440	11	4	91
414	Degermed, enriched:					
	Dry form. . . . . .1 cup	138	500	11	2	108
415	Cooked. . . . . .1 cup	240	120	3	1	26
416	Degermed, unenriched:					
	Dry form. . . . . .1 cup	138	500	11	2	108
417	Cooked. . . . . .1 cup	240	120	3	1	26
418	Corn muffins, made with enriched degermed cornmeal and enriched flour; muffin 2⅜-in. diam.	1 muffin	40	125	3	4	19
419	Corn muffins, made with mix, egg, and milk; muffin 2⅜-in. diam.	1 muffin	40	130	3	4	20
420	Corn, puffed, presweet-ened, added nutrients.	1 cup	30	115	1	Trace	27
421	Corn, shredded, added nutrients.	1 cup	25	100	2	Trace	22
	Crackers:					
422	Graham, 2½-in. square.	4 crackers	28	110	2	3	21
423	Saltines.	4 crackers	11	50	1	1	8
	Danish pastry, plain (without fruit or nuts):					
424	Packaged ring, 12 ounces	1 ring	340	1,435	25	80	155
425	Round piece, approx. 4¼-in. diam. by 1 in.	1 pastry	65	275	5	15	30
426	Ounce . . . . .1 oz.	28	120	2	7	13
427	Doughnuts, cake type . . . .1 doughnut . . .	32	125	1	6	16
428	Farina, quick-cooking, enriched, cooked.	1 cup	245	105	3	Trace	22
	Macaroni, cooked: Enriched:					
429	Cooked, firm stage . . . .1 cup . . . . . . (undergoes additional cooking in a food mixture).		130	190	6	1	39
430	Cooked until tender . . .1 cup	140	155	5	1	32

Food, approximate measure, and weight (in grams)			Calorie	Protein	Fat	Carbo-hydrate
GRAIN PRODUCTS		*Grams*	*Grams*	*Grams*	*Grams*	*Grams*
Unenriched:						
431	Cooked, firm stage . . . .1 cup	130	190	6	1	39
	(undergoes additional cooking in a food mixture).					
432	Cooked until tender . . .1 cup	140	155	5	1	32
433	Macaroni (enriched) and 1 cup	200	430	17	22	40
	cheese, baked.					
434	Canned . . . . .1 cup	240	230	9	10	26
435	Muffins, with enriched 1 muffin	40	120	3	4	17
	white flour; muffin, 3-in. diam.					
	Noodles (egg noodles), cooked:					
436	Enriched . . . . .1 cup	160	200	7	2	37
437	Unenriched . . . . .1 cup	160	200	7	2	37
438	Oats (with or without 1 cup	25	100	3	1	19
	corn) puffed, added nutrients.					
439	Oatmeal or rolled oats, 1 cup	240	130	5	2	23
	cooked.					
	Pancakes, 4-inch diam.:					
440	Wheat, enriched flour 1 cake	27	60	2	2	9
	(home recipe).					
441	Buckwheat (made from 1 cake	27	55	2	2	6
	mix with egg and milk).					
442	Plain or buttermilk 1 cake	27	60	2	2	9
	(made from mix with egg and milk).					
	Pie (piecrust made with unenriched flour):					
	Sector, 4-in., $\frac{1}{7}$ of 9-in. diam. pie:					
443	Apple (2-crust) . . . . . . .1 sector.	135	350	3	15	51
444	Butterscotch (1-crust) . . .1 sector.	130	350	6	14	50
445	Cherry (2-crust). . . . . . .1 sector.	135	350	4	15	52
446	Custard (1-crust) . . . . . .1 sector.	130	285	8	14	30
447	Lemon meringue 1 sector.	120	305	4	12	45
	(1-crust)					
448	Mince (2-crust) . . . . . . .1 sector.	135	365	3	16	56
449	Pecan (1-crust) . . . . . . .1 sector.	118	490	6	27	60
450	Pineapple chiffon 1 sector.	93	265	6	11	36
	(1-crust)					
451	Pumpkin (1-crust). . . . .1 sector.	130	275	5	15	32
	Piecrust, baked shell for pie made with:					
452	Enriched flour. . . . . . . .1 shell	180	900	11	60	79
453	Unenriched flour . . . . . .1 shell	180	900	11	60	79
	Piecrust mix including stick form:					
454	Package, 10-oz., for 1 pkg..	284	1,480	20	93	141
	double crust.					

Food, approximate measure, and weight (in grams)			Calorie	Protein	Fat	Carbo-hydrate

GRAIN PRODUCTS

			Grams	Grams	Grams	Grams	Grams
455	Pizza (cheese) 5½-in. sector; ⅛ of 14-in. diam. pie	1 sector.	75	185	7	6	27
	Popcorn, popped:						
456	Plain, large kernel.	1 cup	6	25	1	Trace	5
457	With oil and salt.	1 cup	9	40	1	2	5
458	Sugar coated.	1 cup	35	135	2	1	30
	Pretzels:						
459	Dutch, twisted.	1 pretzel	16	60	2	1	12
460	Thin, twisted	1 pretzel	6	25	1	Trace	5
461	Stick, small, 2¼ inches . . .	10 sticks	3	10	Trace	Trace	2
462	Stick, regular, 3⅛ inches .	5 sticks.	3	10	Trace	Trace	2
	Rice, white:						
	Enriched:						
463	Raw.	1 cup	185	670	12	1	149
464	Cooked.	1 cup	205	225	4	Trace	50
465	Instant, ready-to-serve.	1 cup	165	180	4	Trace	40
466	Unenriched, cooked . . .	1 cup	205	225	4	Trace	50
467	Parboiled, cooked.	1 cup	175	185	4	Trace	41
468	Rice, puffed, added nutrients.	1 cup	15	60	1	Trace	13
	Rolls, enriched:						
	Cloverleaf or pan:						
469	Home recipe.	1 roll	35	120	3	3	20
470	Commercial	1 roll	28	85	2	2	15
471	Frankfurter or hamburger.	1 roll	40	120	3	2	21
472	Hard, round or rectangular.	1 roll	50	155	5	2	30
473	Rye wafers, whole-grain, 1⅞ by 3½ inches.	2 wafers	13	45	2	Trace	10
474	Spaghetti, cooked, tender stage,	1 cup	140	155	5	1	32
	enriched with meat balls, and tomato sauce:						
475	Home recipe.	1 cup	248	330	19	12	39
476	Canned.	1 cup	250	260	12	10	28
	Spaghetti in tomato sauce with cheese:						
477	Home recipe.	1 cup	250	260	9	9	37
478	Canned.	1 cup	250	190	6	2	38
479	Waffles, with enriched flour, 7-in. diam.	1 waffle	75	210	7	7	28
480	Waffles, made from mix, enriched, egg and milk added, 7-in. diam.	1 waffle	75	205	7	8	27
481	Wheat, puffed, added nutrients.	1 cup	15	55	2	Trace	12

Food, approximate measure, and weight (in grams)			Calorie	Protein	Fat	Carbohydrate
GRAIN PRODUCTS		*Grams*	*Grams*	*Grams*	*Grams*	*Grams*
482 Wheat, shredded, plain	1 biscuit	25	90	2	1	20
483 Wheat flakes, added nutrients.	1 cup	30	105	3	Trace	24
Wheat flours:						
484 Whole-wheat, from hard wheats, stirred.	1 cup	120	400	16	2	85
All-purpose or family flour, enriched:						
485 Sifted.	1 cup	115	420	12	1	88
486 Unsifted	1 cup	125	455	13	1	95
487 Self-rising, enriched.	1 cup	125	440	12	1	93
488 Cake or pastry flour, sifted.	1 cup	96	350	7	1	76
FATS, OILS						
Butter:						
Regular, 4 sticks per pound:						
489 Stick	½ cup	113	810	1	92	1
490 Tablespoon (approx. ⅛ stick).	1 tbsp.	14	100	Trace	12	Trace
491 Pat (1-in. sq. ⅓-in. high; 90 per lb.).	1 pat	5	35	Trace	4	Trace
Whipped, 6 sticks or 2, 8-oz. containers per pound:						
492 Stick	½ cup	76	540	1	61	Trace
493 Tablespoon (approx. ⅛ stick).	1 tbsp.	9	65	Trace	8	Trace
494 Pat (1¼-in. sq. ⅓-in. high; 120 per lb.).	1 pat	4	25	Trace	3	Trace
Fats, cooking:						
495 Lard	1 cup	205	1,850	0	205	0
496	1 tbsp.	13	115	0	13	0
497 Vegetable fat	1 cup	200	1,770	0	200	0
498	1 tbsp.	13	110	0	13	0
Margarine:						
Regular, 4 sticks per pound:						
499 Stick . . . . : .	½ cup	113	815	1	92	1
500 Tablespoon (approx. ⅛ stick).	1 tbsp.	14	100	Trace	12	Trace
501 Pat (1-in. sq. ⅓-in. high; 90 per lb.).	1 pat	5	35	Trace	4	Trace
Whipped, 6 sticks per pound:						
502 Stick	½ cup	76	545	1	61	Trace
Soft, 2 8-oz. tubs per pound:						
503 Tub.	1 tub	227	1,635	1	184	1
504 Tablespoon	1 tbsp.	14	100	Trace	11	Trace

Food, approximate measure, and weight (in grams)		Calorie	Protein	Fat	Carbo-hydrate
FATS, OILS	*Grams*	*Grams*	*Grams*	*Grams*	*Grams*
Oils, salad or cooking:					
505 Corn . . . . .1 cup	220	1,945	0	220	0
506 1 tbsp.	14	125	0	14	0
507 Cottonseed. . . . . .1 cup	220	1,945	0	220	0
508 1 tbsp.	14	125	0	14	0
509 Olive . . . . .1 cup	220	1,945	0	220	0
510 1 tbsp.	14	125	0	14	0
511 Peanut . . . . .1 cup	220	1,945	0	220	0
512 1 tbsp.	14	125	0	14	0
513 Safflower. . . . . .1 cup	220	1,945	0	220	0
514 1 tbsp.	14	125	0	14	0
515 Soybean . . . . .1 cup	220	1,945	0	220	0
516 1 tbsp.	14	125	0	14	0
Salad dressings:					
517 Blue cheese . . . . .1 tbsp.	15	75	1	8	1
Commercial, mayonnaise type:					
518 Regular. . . . . .1 tbsp.	15	65	Trace	6	2
519 Special dietary, low- 1 tbsp. . . . . . . calorie.	16	20	Trace	2	1
French:					
520 Regular. . . . . .1 tbsp.	16	65	Trace	6	3
521 Special dietary, low- 1 tbsp. . . . . . . fat with artificial sweeteners.	15	Trace	Trace	Trace	Trace
522 Home cooked, boiled. . .1 tbsp.	16	25	1	2	2
523 Mayonnaise . . . . .1 tbsp.	14	100	Trace	11	Trace
524 Thousand island. . . . . .1 tbsp.	16	80	Trace	8	3
SUGARS, SWEETS					
Cake icing:					
525 Chocolate made with 1 cup . . . . milk and table fat.	275	1,035	9	38	185
526 Coconut (with boiled 1 cup . . . . icing).	166	605	3	13	124
527 Creamy fudge from 1 cup . . . . mix with water only.	245	830	7	16	183
528 White, boiled . . . . . . .1 cup	94	300	1	0	76
Candy:					
529 Caramels, plain or 1 oz. . . . . chocolate.	28	115	1	3	22
530 Chocolate, milk, plain . . .1 oz.	28	145	2	9	16
531 Chocolate-coated 1 oz. . . . . peanuts.	28	160	5	12	11
532 Fondant; mints, un- 1 oz. . . . . coated; candy corn.	28	105	Trace	1	25
533 Fudge, plain . . . . .1 oz.	28	115	1	4	21

Food, approximate measure, and weight (in grams)		Calorie	Protein	Fat	Carbo-hydrate
SUGARS, SWEETS	*Grams*	*Grams*	*Grams*	*Grams*	*Grams*
534 Gum drops. . . . . .1 oz.	28	100	Trace	Trace	25
535 Hard . . . . .1 oz.	28	110	0	Trace	28
536 Marshmallows . . . . .1 oz.	28	90	1	Trace	23
Chocolate-flavoured sirup or topping:					
537 Thin type . . . . .1 fl. oz	38	90	1	1	24
538 Fudge type. . . . . .1 fl. oz	38	125	2	5	20
Chocolate-flavoured beverage powder (approx. 4 heaping teaspoons per oz.):					
539 With nonfat dry milk . . . .1 oz.	28	100	5	1	20
540 Without nonfat dry milk. 1 oz.	28	100	1	1	25
541 Honey, strained or extracted. 1 tbsp.	21	65	Trace	0	17
542 Jam and preserves. . . . . . .1 tbsp.	20	55	Trace	Trace	14
543 Jellies. . . . . .1 tbsp.	18	50	Trace	Trace	13
Molasses, cane:					
544 Light (first extraction) . . .1 tbsp.	20	50	–	–	13
545 Blackstrap (third extraction). 1 tbsp.	20	45	–	–	11
Sirups:					
546 Sorghum . . . . .1 tbsp.	21	55	–	–	14
547 Table blends, chiefly corn, light and dark. 1 tbsp.	21	60	0	0	15
Sugars:					
548 Brown, firm packed. . . . .1 cup	220	820	0	0	212
White:					
549 Granulated. . . . . .1 cup	200	770	0	0	199
550 1 tbsp.	11	40	0	0	11
551 Powdered, stirred before measuring. 1 cup	120	460	0	0	119
MISCELLANEOUS ITEMS					
552 Barbecue sauce . . . . . . .1 cup	250	230	4	17	20
Beverages, alcoholic:					
553 Beer. . . . . .12 fl. oz	360	150	1	0	14
Gin, rum, vodka, whiskey:					
554 80-proof . . . . .1½ fl. oz. jigger.	42	100	–	–	Trace
555 86-proof . . . . .1½ fl. oz. jigger.	42	105	–	–	Trace
556 90-proof . . . . .1½ fl. oz. jigger.	42	110	–	–	Trace
557 94-proof . . . . .1½ fl. oz. jigger.	42	115			Trace
558 100-proof 1½ fl. oz. jigger.	42	125		. . . .	.Trace

	Food, approximate measure, and weight (in grams)		Calorie	Protein	Fat	Carbo-hydrate
	MISCELLANEOUS ITEMS		*Grams*	*Grams*	*Grams*	*Grams* *Grams*
	Wines:					
559	Dessert . . . . .3½ fl. oz. glass.	103	140	Trace	0	8
560	Table . . . . .3½ fl. oz. glass.	102	85	Trace	0	4
	Beverages, carbonated, sweetened, nonalcoholic:					
561	Carbonated water. . . . . .12 fl. oz	366	115	0	0	29
562	Cola type. . . . . .12 fl. oz	369	145	0	0	37
563	Fruit-flavoured sodas. . . .12 fl. oz . . . . . and Tom Collins mixes	372	170	0	0	45
564	Ginger ale . . . . .12 fl. oz	366	115	0	0	29
565	Root beer . . . . .12 fl. oz	370	150	0	0	39
566	Bouillon cubes, approx. 1 cube . . . . . . ½ in.	4	5	1	Trace	Trace
	Chocolate:					
567	Bitter or baking . . . . . . .1 oz.	28	145	3	15	8
568	Semi-sweet, small 1 cup . . . . pieces.	170	860	7	61	97
	Gelatin:					
569	Plain, dry powder in 1 envelope . . . . envelope.	7	25	6	Trace	0
570	Dessert powder, 3-oz. 1 pkg . . . . package.	85	315	8	0	75
571	Gelatin dessert, prepared 1 cup . . . . . . with water.	240	140	4	0	34
	Olives, pickled:					
572	Green. . . . . .4 medium or 3 extra large or 2 giant.	16	15	Trace	2	Trace
573	Ripe: Mission . . . . . . .3 small or 2 large.	10	15	Trace	2	Trace
	Pickles, cucumber:					
574	Dill, medium, whole, 1 pickle. . . . . . 3¾ in. long, 1¼ in. diam.	65	10	1	Trace	1
575	Fresh, sliced, 1½ in. 2 slices . . . . . . diam. ¼ in. thick.	15	10	Trace	Trace	3
576	Sweet, gherkin, small, 1 pickle. . . . . . whole, approx. 2½ in. long, ¾ in. diam.	15	20	Trace	Trace	6
577	Relish, finely chopped, 1 tbsp. . . . . . . sweet.	15	20	Trace	Trace	5
	Popcorn. See Grain Products.					
578	Popsicle, 3 fl. oz. size. . . . .1 popsicle	95	70	0	0	18
	Pudding, home recipe with starch base:					
579	Chocolate . . . . .1 cup	260	385	8	12	67
580	Vanilla (blancmange). . . .1 cup	255	285	9	10	41

Food, approximate measure, and weight (in grams)			Caloric	Protein	Fat	Carbo-hydrate
MISCELLANEOUS ITEMS		*Grams*	*Grams*	*Grams*	*Grams*	*Grams*
581	Pudding mix, dry form, 4-oz package.	1 pkg 113	410	3	2	103
582	Sherbet. . . . . .1 cup 193		260	2	2	59
	Soups:					
	Canned, condensed, ready-to-serve:					
	Prepared with an equal volume of milk:					
583	Cream of chicken . . . .1 cup 245		180	7	10	15
584	Cream of mushroom . .1 cup 245		215	7	14	16
585	Tomato. . . . . .1 cup 250		175	7	7	23
	Prepared with an equal volume of water:					
586	Bean with pork . . . . .1 cup 250		170	8	6	22
587	Beef broth, bouillon consomme.	1 cup 240	30	5	0	3
588	Beef noodle . . . . . . .1 cup 240		70	4	3	7
589	Clam chowder, Manhattan type (with tomatoes, without milk).	1 cup 245	80	2	3	12
590	Cream of chicken . . . .1 cup 240		95	3	6	8
591	Cream of mushroom . .1 cup 240		135	2	10	10
592	Minestrone. . . . . . . .1 cup 245		105	5	3	14
593	Split pea . . . . .1 cup 245		145	9	3	21
594	Tomato. . . . . .1 cup 245		90	2	3	16
595	Vegetable beef. . . . . .1 cup 245		80	5	2	10
596	Vegetarian . . . . .1 cup 245		80	2	2	13
	Dehydrated, dry form:					
597	Chicken noodle (2-oz. package).	1 pkg 57	220	8	6	33
598	Onion mix (1½-oz. package).	1 pkg 43	150	6	5	23
599	Tomato vegetable with noodles (2½-oz pkg).	1 pkg 71	245	6	6	45
	Frozen, condensed:					
	Clam chowder, New England type (with milk, without tomatoes):					
600	Prepared with equal volume of milk.	1 cup 245	210	9	12	16
601	Prepared with equal volume of water.	1 cup 240	130	4	8	11
	Cream of potato:					
602	Prepared with equal volume of milk.	1 cup 245	185	8	10	18
603	Prepared with equal volume of water.	1 cup 240	105	3	5	12
	Cream of shrimp:					
604	Prepared with equal volume of milk.	1 cup 245	245	9	16	15

Food, approximate measure, and weight (in grams)			Calorie	Protein	Fat	Carbo-hydrate
MISCELLANEOUS ITEMS			*Grams*	*Grams*	*Grams*	*Grams* *Grams*
605	Prepared with equal volume of water.	1 cup	240	160	5	12	8
	Oyster stew:					
606	Prepared with equal volume of milk.	1 cup	240	200	10	12	14
607	Prepared with equal volume of water.	1 cup	240	120	6	8	8
608	Tapioca, dry, quick-cooking	1 cup	152	535	1	Trace	131
	Tapioca desserts:					
609	Apple.	1 cup	250	295	1	Trace	74
610	Cream pudding	1 cup	165	220	8	8	28
611	Tartar sauce	1 tbsp.	14	75	Trace	8	1
612	Vinegar.	1 tbsp.	15	Trace	Trace	0	1
613	White sauce, medium	1 cup	250	405	10	31	22
	Yeast:					
614	Baker's, dry, active	1 pkg	7	20	3	Trace	3
615	Brewer's, dry	1 tbsp.	8	25	3	Trace	3
	Yoghurt. See Milk, Cheese, Cream, Imitation Cream.					

APPENDIX D

A list of conditions which may either preclude exercise or call for a great deal more caution. Only your doctor is in a position to evaluate these 'contraindications' to exercise. (Source: *Guidelines for Graded Exercise Testing and Exercise Prescription*, American College of Sport Medicine, Lea and Febiger, Philadelphia, 1975.)

Absolute Contraindications	'Translation'[1]
1 Congestive heart failure	The heart is not keeping up with its work load resulting in an increased venous return causing a backup of fluids.
2 Acute myocardial infarction	A recent heart attack in which a portion of the heart has died.
3 Active myocarditis	An inflammation of the heart wall.
4 Rapidly increasing angina pectoris with effort	Severe chest pains (sometimes spreading to the arms and up the neck) which are getting worse, with any type of physical work.
5 Recent embolism, either systemic or pulmonary	A foreign body, usually a blood clot, in the blood stream which can obstruct a small blood vessel.
6 Dissecting aneurysm	Progressive dilation and destruction of a blood vessel wall.

[1] In consultation with David Hammond, M.D. of Ithaca College we have attempted to describe these terms for the layman.

Absolute Contraindications	'Translation'[1]
7 Thrombophlebitis	Inflammation of the veins with clot formation.
8 Acute infectious disease	Presence of active infectious disease.
9 Ventricular tachycardia	A serious electrocardiogram abnormality which is characterized by rapidly contracting ventricles (220/min).
10 Severe aortic stenosis	The valves in the opening from the left ventricle to the aorta are calcified (hardened) and constricted thus severely narrowing the opening.

Relative Contraindications

1 Uncontrolled or high-rate supraventricular dysrhythmia	An abnormal electrocardiogram.
2 Repetitive or frequent ventricular ectopic activity	An abnormal electrocardiogram.
3 Untreated severe systemic or pulmonary hypertension	Untreated high blood pressure, in the system or in the lungs.
4 Ventricular aneurysm	A blood filled sac formed by the dilation or expansion of part of an artery.
5 Moderate aortic stenosis	Less serious than the severe aortic stenosis described above. Less constricted opening.
6 Uncontrolled metabolic disease (diabetes, thyrotoxicosis, myxedema)	Describes itself.
7 Marked cardiac enlargement	Increase in size and thickness of ventricular walls without accompanying collateral circulation.
8 Toxemia of pregnancy	A pathological condition occurring in pregnant women characterized by the presence in the blood of certain toxic products.

Conditions Requiring Special Consideration and/or Precaution

1 Conduction disturbances
  a) Complete AV block
  b) Left bundle branch block
  c) Wolff-Parkinson-White
    syndrome
	Abnormalities in the electrocardiogram.

2 Fixed rate pacemaker	Presence of an artificial pacemaker which performs the function of a normal heart in fixing the normal resting rate of heart contractions.
3 Certain medication, for example, Digitalis or Beta-Blocking Drugs	Commonly used drugs which strengthen the heart resulting in a much slower exercise and resting heart rate.
4 Clinically severe hypertension (Diastoli over 110, grade III retinopathy)	High blood pressure.
5 Angina Pectoris	Stable chest pain as described above.
6 Cyanotic Heart Disease	Failure of blood oxygenation process resulting in a lack of oxygen to the body.
7 Severe Anaemia	Decrease in red blood cells, haemoglobin or both.
8 Marked Obesity	Over thirty to thirty-five per cent body fat.
9 Renal, hepatic and other metabolic insufficiency	Abnormalities of such organs as the kidney or liver.
10 Overt Psychoneurotic disturbance requiring therapy	Certain types of mental illness.
11 Neuromuscular, musculoskeletal or arthritic disorders which would prevent activity	Explains itself.

Adams, C.F.,   *Nutritive Value of American Foods*, Agriculture Handbook, No 456, USDA, November, 1975.

American College of Sports Medicine,   *Guidelines for Graded Exercise Testing and Exercise Prescription* Philadelphia: Lea and Febiger, 1976.

American College of Sports Medicine,   'Position Statement on the recommended quantity of quality of exercise for developing and maintaining fitness in healthy adults.' *Medicine and Science in Sports* 10: vii–x, 1978.

Åstrand, P.O. and Rodahl, K.,   *Textbook of Work Physiology* (2nd Edition) New York: McGraw Hill Co., 1977.

Åstrand, P.O.,   'Do we need physical conditioning?' *Journal of Physical Education*, 129–136, March–April, 1972.

Attenborough, D.,   *Life on Earth* London: William Collins Sons and Co. Ltd, 1979.

Bellamy, D.,   *Botanic Man* London: Hamlyn Publishing, 1978.

Benesetad, A.M.,   'Trainability of Old Men', *Acta. Med. Scand.* 178: 321–327, 1965.

Berger, R.,   'Effect of Varied Weight Training Program on Strength' *Research Quarterly*, 33: 168, 1962.

Bogert, L.J. and Briggs, G.M.,   *Nutrition and Physical Fitness* (9th Edition) Philadelphia: W.B. Saunders, 1973.

Borg, G.,   'The perception of physical performance' In *Frontiers of Fitness*, R.J. Shephard (ed.) Springfield, Illinois: Thomas Co., 1971.

Bronowski, J., *The Ascent of Man* Boston: Little, Brown & Co, 1973.

Burke, E.J., A factor analytic investigation of tests of physical working capacity. *Ergonomics* 22: 11–18, 1979.

Burke, E.J., An Analysis of Physical Fitness. In *Relevant Topics for Athletic Training*. Scriber, K. & Burke, E. (Eds.) Ithaca, N.Y. Mouvement Publications, 1978.

Burke, E.J., Physiological effects of similar training programs in males and females. *Research Quarterly*, 48: 510–517, 1976.

Burke E.J., 'Individualized fitness programme using perceived exertion for the prescription of healthy adults.' *Journal of Physical Education & Recreation*. November, 1979.

Burke, E.J., Work physiology and the components of physical fitness in the analysis of human performance. In: *Toward an Understanding of Human Performance*. Burke, E. (ed.) Ithaca, N.Y.: Mouvement Publications, (2nd Ed. 1980).

Burke, E.J. and Brush, F., Physiological and anthropometric assessment of successful teenage female distance runners *Research Quarterly*. Fall, 1979.

Chapman, C.B. and Mitchell, J.H., 'The physiology of exercise'. *Scientific American*, 212, 5: 88–96, 1965.

Cheffers, J. and Evaul, T., *Introduction to Physical Education* Englewood Cliffs: Prentice-Hall, 1978.

Clarke, D.H., 'Adaptations in strength and muscular endurance resulting from exercise.' *Exercise & Sports Sciences Reviews*, 1, Wilmore, J.H. (ed.) New York: Academic Press, 1973.

Clarke, H.H., *Modern Athlete & Coach* Vol. 11, no. 2, March, 1973.

Clegg, E.J., *The Study of Man*, (2nd Edition), London: Hodder & Stoughton, 1978.

Cohen, D., — Old Age Steals Away Their Brains, *The Listener*, Vol. 103, no. 2646, 24.1. 1980.

Cooper, K.H., — *Aerobics* New York: Bantam Books, 1968.

Cooper, K.H. and Cooper, M., — *Aerobics for Women* New York: Bantam Books, 1972.

Cooper, K.H., Pollock M.L., Martin, R.P., White, S.R., Linnerud, A.C., and Jackson, A., — 'Physical fitness levels vs selected coronary risks factors' *Journal of the American Medical Association.* 236: 166–169, 1976.

Cooper, K., — *The Aerobics Way* London: Corgi Books, 1978.

Cooper, K., — *The New Aerobics* New York: Bantam Books, 1970.

Corbin, C.B., Dowell, L., Lindsay, R. and Tolson, H., — *Concepts in Physical Education with Laboratories and Experiments* Iowa: Wm. C. Brown, 1970.

Davies, C.T.M. and Knibbs, A., — 'The training stimulus the effects of intensity duration and frequency of effort on maximum aerobic power output'. *Int.Z.Angew.* 29: 299–305, 1971.

De Vries, H.A., — *Physiology of Exericse for Physical Education & Athletics* Dubuque, Iowa: W.C. Brown Co. (2nd ed.), 1974.

De Vries, H., — 'Evaluation of static stretching procedures for improvement of flexibility'. *Research Quarterly*, 33: 222–229, 1962.

De Vries, H.A., — 'Exercise intensity threshold for improvement of cardiovascular – respiratory function in older men.' *Geriatrics* 26, 49–101, 1971.

De Vries, H.A., — 'Physiological effects of an exercise training reigmen upon men aged 52–88' *J. Geront.* 25: 325–336, 1970.

Dintiman, G.B., — *'What research tells the coach about sprinting'* Washington: A.A.H.P.E.R. Publications, 1974.

Eccles, J.C., — *The Understanding of the Brain* New York: McGraw Hill, 1973.

Eckstein, R.W., — 'Effect of exercise and coronary artery narrowing on coronary collateral circu-

Eddington, D.W. and Edgerton, V.R.,

Ekblom, B.,

lation of dogs.' *Circ. Res.* 5: 230, 1957.
The Biology of Physical Activity Boston: Houghton Mifflin Co., 1976.
'Effect of physical training on the O_2 transport system in man.' Act. Physiol. Scand. Supp. 328 1969.

Falls, H.B., Wallis, E.L., and Logan, G.A.,

Foundations of Conditioning New York: Academic Press, 1970.

Feldenkrais, M.,

Awareness Through Movement New York: Hayes and Row, 1972.

Feldenkrais, M.,

Body and Mature Behavior New York: International Universities Press Inc, 1949.

Fentem, P.H. and Bassey, E.J.,

'The case for exercise' London: The Sports Council, 1978.

Ferguson, R.J., Petitclerc, R., Choquette, G. et al.,

'Effect of physical training on treadmill exercise capacity, collateral circulation and progression of coronary disease.' *Am.J. Cardiol.* 34: 765, 1974.

Fixx, J.F.,

The Complete Book of Running New York: Random House, 1977.

Fleishman, E.,

The Structure and Measurement of Physical Fitness Englewood Cliffs, N.J.: Prentice-Hall Inc., 1964.

Fox, E.L., Bartels, R.L., Billings, C.E., O'Brien, R., Bason, R., and Matthews, D.K.,

'Frequency and duration of interval training programs and changes in aerobic power.' *J.Appl. Physiol.* 38: 481–484, 1975.

Fox, S.M., Naughton, J.P., and Gorman, P.A.,

'Physical activity and cardio-vascular health,' *Modern Concepts of Cardiovascular Disease.* 16, June, 1972.

Froelicher, V.F.,

'Does exercise conditioning delay progression of myocardial ischemia in coronary atherosclerotic heart disease.' *Cardiovascular Clinics 8*: 11–31, 1977.

Gardner, R.A. and Gardner, B.T.,

'Teaching Sign-Language to a Chimpanzee' *Science* 165: 664–672, 1969.

Getchell, B.,

Physical Fitness A Way of Life New York: John Wiley & Sons, 1976.

Goodall, J.,

'Tool-using and aimed throwing in a community of free-living chimpanzees.' *Nature* 201: 1264–1266, 1964.

Graham, M.F.,

Prescription for Life New York:

Harlow, H.F.,   David McKay Co., 1966.
'Love in infant monkeys.' *Scientific American*, July, 1959.

Harlow, H.F.,   'The nature of love' *American Psychologist*, 12: 673–685, 1958.

Holloway, R.L.,   'The Evolution of the primate brain: some aspects of quantitative relations'. *Brain Research* 7: 121–172, 1968.

Homel, S. and Evaul, T.,   *Understanding Human Behaviour – A Needs Approach* Philadelphia: Temple University, 1968.

Howe, P.S.,   *Basic Nutrition In Health & Disease* Philadelphia: W.B. Saunders, 1971.

Hultgren, P.B. and Burke, E.J.,   'Methodology for prescription of exercise.' *Australian Journal of Sports Medicine* 8, 127–130, 1976.

Humphreys, J.H.L.,   'Cardio-Respiratory Indices of Endurance Capacity in Soccer Players,' *Ph.D. Diss.* Loughborough University, 1977.

Johnson, P., Updyke, W., Schaefer, M. and Stolberg, D.,   *Sport Exercise and You* New York: Holt Rinehart & Winston, 1975.

Jolliffe, N.,   *The Prudent Diet* New York: Simon & Schuster, 1963.

Kasch, F.W.,   'The effects of exercise on the ageing process' *The Physician & Sports Medicine* 64–68 June, 1976.

Katch, F.I. and McArdle, W.D.,   *Nutrition Weight Control and Exercise* Boston: Houghton-Mifflin, 1977.

Kavanaugh, T., Shephard, R.H. and Pandit, V.,   'Marathon running after myocardial infarction'. *Journal of American Medical Association* 229: 162, 1974.

Klissouras, V.,   'Adaptability of genetic variation.' *Journal of Applied Physiology*, 31: 338–344, 1971.

Knehr, C.A., Dill, D.B., and Neufeld, W.,   'Training and its effects on man at rest and at work.' *Amer.J. Physiol.* 136: 148–156, 1942.

Lamb, D.,   'Androgens and exercise.' *Medicine & Science in Sport*, 7: 1–5, 1975.

Lamb, D.R.,   *Physiology of Exercise* New York: MacMillan, 1978.

Leakey, R.E.F. and Walker, A.C.,   'Australopithecus, Homo Erectus and the single species hypothesis.' *Nature* 261: 572–574, 1976.

Lowenberg, M., Todhunter, E., Wilson, E., Savage, J., Lubanski, J., MacLean, P., *Food and Man* New York: John Wiley & Son, 1974.

A Triune Concept of the Brain and Behaviour Toronto: University of Toronto Press, 1973.

Matthews, D.K. and Fox, E.L., *The Physiological Basis of Physical Education and Athletics* Philadelphia: W.B. Saunders Co., 1967.

Mayer, J., 'Nutrition's future: food for thought.' *Family Health* 7: 42, January 1975.

Mayer, J., *Overweight Causes Cost and Control* Englewood Cliffs: Prentice Hall, 1968.

Mayer, J., 'When you think food, think the basic seven.' *Family Health* 7: 27, September 1974.

Michael, E., Burke, E. and Avakion, E., *Laboratory Experiences in Exercise Physiology* Ithaca, N.Y.: Mouvement Publications, 1979.

Morehouse, L.E. and Miller, A.T., *Physiology of Exercise* (7th Edition) St Louis: C.V. Mosby, 1976.

Oja, P., Teraslinna, P., Partaner, T. and Karava, R., 'Feasibility of an 18 months' physical training programme for middle-aged men and its effect on physical fitness.' *Am.J.Public Health* 64: 459–465, 1975.

O'Shea, J.P., *Scientific Principles and Methods of Strength Fitness* (2nd Edition), Reading Mass: Addison Wesley C., 1976.

Oxmard, C.E., 'The place of the oustralopithecines in human evolution: grounds for doubt?' *Nature* 258: 389–395, 1975.

Pollock, M.L., 'Now much exercise is enough?' *The Physician and Sportsmedicine* 6: June, 1978.

Pollock, M.L., Miller, H.S., Linnerud, A.C. and Cooper, K.H., 'Frequency of training as a determinant for improvement in cardiovascular function and body composition of middle-aged men.' *Arch.Phys.Med. Rehab.* 56: 141–145, 1975.

Pollock, M.L., Wilmore, J.H. and Fox, S.M.III., *Health & Fitness Through Physical Activity* New York: John Wiley & Sons, 1978.

Presidents Council on 'National adult physical fitness survey'

Physical Fitness and Sports, Raab, W., Newsletter PCPFS, May 1973. *Prevention Myocardology* Springfield, Ill: Charles C. Thomas Co., 1970.

Radinsky, L., 'Primate brain evolution.' *American Scientist* 63: 656–663, 1975.

Rockefeller, K. and Burke, E., 'Psycho-physiological analysis of an aerobic dance programme for women.' *British Journal of Sports Medicine*, 13, 77–80, 1979.

Runner's World Editors, *The Complete Runner* Mountainview, Cal: World Publications, 1974.

Sachs, M. and Pargman, D., '*Addiction to running*: phenomon or pseudo-phenomonon?' Paper presented at the International Congress in Physical Education, Université du Québec à Trois-Riviéres, June, 1979.

Sagan, C., *The Dragons of Eden* New York: Ballantine Books, 1977.

Saltin, B., 'Physiological effects of physical conditioning.' *Medicine and Science In Sports* 1, March, 1969.

Saltin, B.L., Hartley, L. Kilborn, A. and Astrand, I., 'Physical training in sedentary middle-aged and older men.' *Scand.J.Clin.Lab. Invest.* 24: 323–334. 1969.

Sharkey, B.J., *Physiology of Fitness* Champaign, Ill: Human Kinetics, 1979.

Sharkey, B.J., *Physiology and Physical Activity* New York: Harper & Row, 1975.

Shephard, R.J., *Physical Activity and Ageing* Chicago: Year Book Medical Publishers, 1978.

Tepperman, J. and Pearlman, D., 'Effects of exercise and anaemia on coronary arteries of small animals as revealed by the corrosion-cast technique.' *Circ.Res.* 9: 576, 1961.

Thomas, L., *The Medusa and the Snail* New York: Viking Press, 1979.

Thomas, L., *The Lives of a Cell* New York: Viking Press, 1973.

Tiger, L., 'A very old animal called man.' *Newsweek*, Sept, 4, 1978.

Tomanek, R.J., 'Effects of age and exercise on the extent of myocardial capillary bed.' *Anat.Rec.* 167: 55, 1970.

U.S.D.H.E.W., 'Nutrition nonsense – and sense.' *FDA*

Van Huss, W.D.,   *Fact Sheet* Rockville, Maryland: Food and Drug Administration, July, 1971. 'Physical Activity and Ageing' *Sports Medicine & Physiology* Straus, R.H. (ed.) Philadelphia: W.B. Saunders, 1979.

White, P.L., (ed.).,   *Let's Talk About Food* Chicago: American Medical Association, 1970.

Wilmore, J.,   *Athletic Training and Physical Fitness* Boston: Allyn & Bacon, 1976.

Wilmore, J.,   Alterations in strength, body composition and anthropometric measurements consequent to a 10 week weight training program. *Med.Sci.Sport* 6, 133–138, 1974.

Wilmore, J.,   'Individual exercise prescription.' *The American Journal of Cardiology* 33: 757–759, 1974.

Wolf, J.,   *The Dawn of Man* London: Thames and Hudson, 1978.

Young, J.Z.,   *An Introduction to the Study of Man* London: Oxford University Press, 1974.